MW00845873

Drug Development for Rare Diseases

A disease is defined as rare if the prevalence is fewer than 200,000 in the United States. It is estimated that there are more than 7,000 rare diseases, which collectively affect 30 million Americans or 10% of the US population. This diverse and complex disease area poses challenges for patients, caregivers, regulators, drug developers, and other stakeholders. This book is proposed to give an overview of the common issues facing rare disease drug developers, summarize challenges specific to clinical development in small populations, discuss drug development strategies in the evolving regulatory environment, explain generation and utilization of different data and evidence inside and beyond clinical trials, and use recent examples to demonstrate these challenges and the development strategies that respond to the challenges.

Key Features:

- Rare disease.
- Drug development.
- Innovative clinical trial design.
- Regulatory approval.
- Real-world evidence.

Chapman & Hall/CRC Biostatistics Series

Series Editors:
Shein-Chung Chow, Duke University School of Medicine, USA
Byron Jones, Novartis Pharma AG, Switzerland
Jen-pei Liu, National Taiwan University, Taiwan
Karl E. Peace, Georgia Southern University, USA
Bruce W. Turnbull, Cornell University, USA

RECENTLY PUBLISHED TITLES

Real World Evidence in a Patient-Centric Digital Era
Edited by Kelly H. Zou, Lobna A. Salem, and Amrit Ray

Data Science, AI, and Machine Learning in Pharma
Harry Yang

Model-Assisted Bayesian Designs for Dose Finding and Optimization
Methods and Applications
Ying Yuan, Ruitao Lin, and J. Jack Lee

Digital Therapeutics: Strategic, Scientific, Developmental, and Regulatory Aspects
Oleksandr Sverdlov and Joris van Dam

Quantitative Methods for Precision Medicine
Pharmacogenomics in Action
Rongling Wu

Drug Development for Rare Diseases
Edited by Bo Yang, Yang Song, and Yijie Zhou

Case Studies in Bayesian Methods for Biopharmaceutical CMC
Edited by Paul Faya and Tony Pourmohamad

Statistical Analytics for Health Data Science with SAS and R
Jeffrey Wilson, Ding-Geng Chen, and Karl E. Peace

For more information about this series, please visit: https://www.routledge.com/Chapman—Hall-CRC-Biostatistics-Series/book-series/CHBIOSTATIS

Drug Development for Rare Diseases

Edited by
Bo Yang, Yang Song, and Yijie Zhou

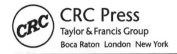

CRC Press
Taylor & Francis Group
Boca Raton London New York

CRC Press is an imprint of the
Taylor & Francis Group, an **informa** business

A CHAPMAN & HALL BOOK

First edition published 2023
by CRC Press
6000 Broken Sound Parkway NW, Suite 300, Boca Raton, FL 33487-2742

and by CRC Press
4 Park Square, Milton Park, Abingdon, Oxon, OX14 4RN

CRC Press is an imprint of Taylor & Francis Group, LLC

© 2023 Taylor & Francis Group, LLC

Reasonable efforts have been made to publish reliable data and information, but the author and publisher cannot assume responsibility for the validity of all materials or the consequences of their use. The authors and publishers have attempted to trace the copyright holders of all material reproduced in this publication and apologize to copyright holders if permission to publish in this form has not been obtained. If any copyright material has not been acknowledged please write and let us know so we may rectify in any future reprint.

Except as permitted under U.S. Copyright Law, no part of this book may be reprinted, reproduced, transmitted, or utilized in any form by any electronic, mechanical, or other means, now known or hereafter invented, including photocopying, microfilming, and recording, or in any information storage or retrieval system, without written permission from the publishers.

For permission to photocopy or use material electronically from this work, access www.copyright.com or contact the Copyright Clearance Center, Inc. (CCC), 222 Rosewood Drive, Danvers, MA 01923, 978-750-8400. For works that are not available on CCC please contact mpkbookspermissions@tandf.co.uk

Trademark notice: Product or corporate names may be trademarks or registered trademarks and are used only for identification and explanation without intent to infringe.

ISBN: 9780367518349 (hbk)
ISBN: 9780367532116 (pbk)
ISBN: 9781003080954 (ebk)

DOI: 10.1201/9781003080954

Typeset in Palatino
by codeMantra

Contents

Editors

Bo Yang is the Vice President, Biometrics and Real World Evidence at Vertex Pharmaceuticals, USA.

Yang Song is the Executive Director, Biostatistics Group Head of Pipeline Development at Vertex Pharmaceuticals, USA.

Yijie Zhou is the Executive Director, Real World Statistics and Analytics at Vertex Pharmaceuticals, USA.

Contributors

Amy Barone
Office of Oncologic Diseases (OOD),
  Office of New Drugs, Center for
  Drug Evaluation and Research
  (CDER)
US Food and Drug Administration
Silver Spring, Maryland

Brenda Cirincione
Clinical and Quantitative
  Pharmacology
Vertex Pharmaceuticals
Boston, MA

Charu Gandotra
Office of Cardiology, Hematology,
  Endocrinology and Nephrology
  (OCHEN), Office of New Drugs,
  Center for Drug Evaluation and
  Research (CDER)
US Food and Drug Administration
  (FDA)
Silver Spring, Maryland

Ina Jazic
Biometrics & Real World Evidence
Vertex Pharmaceuticals
Boston, Massachusetts

Glen Laird
Biometrics & Real World Evidence
Vertex Pharmaceuticals
Boston, Massachusetts

Kerry Jo Lee
Office of Rare Diseases, Pediatrics,
  Urologic and Reproductive
  Medicine (ORPURM), Office of
  New Drugs, Center for Drug
  Evaluation and Research (CDER)
US Food and Drug Administration
Silver Spring, Maryland

Lingyun Liu
Biometrics & Real World Evidence
Vertex Pharmaceuticals
Boston, Massachusetts

Tina Liu
Biometrics & Real World Evidence
Vertex Pharmaceuticals
Boston, Massachusetts

Xiaoyan Liu
Biometrics & Real World Evidence
Vertex Pharmaceuticals
Boston, Massachusetts

Yimeng Lu
Biometrics
Vir Biotechnology
San Francisco, California

Xiaolong Luo
Biometrics
Sarepta Pharmaceuticals
Cambridge, Massachusetts

Lian Ma
Division of Pharmacometrics, Office
of Clinical Pharmacology, Center
for Drug Evaluation and Research
(CDER)
US Food and Drug Administration
Silver Spring, Maryland

Xiaopeng Miao
Biometrics & Real World Evidence
Vertex Pharmaceuticals
Boston, Massachusetts

Nitin Nair
Biometrics & Real World Evidence
Vertex Pharmaceuticals
Boston, Massachusetts

Joanne Palmisano
Regulatory Affairs and Global
Regulatory Strategy
Vertex Pharmaceuticals (now
retired)
Boston, Massachusetts

Mark Peterson
Clinical and Quantitative
Pharmacology
Vertex Pharmaceuticals
Boston, Massachusetts

Nicholas Richardson
Office of Oncologic Diseases (OOD),
Office of New Drugs, Center for
Drug Evaluation and Research
(CDER)
US Food and Drug Administration
Silver Spring, Maryland

Lina Titievsky
Biometrics & Real World Evidence
Vertex Pharmaceuticals
Boston, Massachusetts

Nataliya Volkova
Global Patient Safety Epidemiology
Vertex Pharmaceuticals
Boston, Massachusetts

Chenkun Wang
Biometrics & Real World Evidence
Vertex Pharmaceuticals
Boston, Massachusetts

Emily Wearne
Office of Oncologic Diseases (OOD),
Office of New Drugs, Center for
Drug Evaluation and Research
(CDER)
US Food and Drug Administration
Silver Spring, Maryland

Tu Xu
Biometrics & Real World Evidence
Vertex Pharmaceuticals
Boston, Massachusetts

Jingjing Ye
Global Statistics and Data Science
(GSDS)
BeiGene
Fulton, Maryland

Bingming Yi
Biometrics & Real World Evidence
Vertex Pharmaceuticals
Boston, Massachusetts

Jason Yuan
Biometrics
Neumora Therapeutics
Watertown, Massachusetts

Lanju Zhang
Biometrics & Real World Evidence
Vertex Pharmaceuticals
Boston, Massachusetts

1

Introduction to Rare Disease Therapy Development

Glen Laird

Vertex Pharmaceuticals

CONTENTS

1.1 Introduction

> Plus ça change
> Plus ç'est la même chose
> (The more that things change
> The more they stay the same)
>
> **~ Jean-Baptiste Alphonse Karr (1808–1890)**

The circumstance of medicine for rare diseases has been described as both rapidly developing and unchanging. Both descriptions have merit. There are approximately 7,000 known rare diseases (Haendel et al., 2020; National Institutes of Health, 2020), and certain commonalities emerge. Many of these rare diseases are genetic in origin, with 80% thought to have an identified genetic cause, resulting in most (50%~75%) of the patients being children (Wright et al., 2018). There is no explicit international definition of a serious disease, but typically, many rare diseases are quite severe, even life-threatening or life-shortening, in nature. Therefore, a clinical expectation of a gradual patient decline (with varying timeframe) is antici-pated. Therapeutic progress has been dramatic (Miller et al., 2021), with exciting principles established, in selected areas such as chronic myeloid leukemia, spinal muscular atrophy, and cystic fibrosis. For example, the 5-year survival rate for chronic myeloid leukemia, previously about 30%, has been cited as at least 89% since the advent of imatinib therapy target-ing the genetic source of the disorder, the BCR-ABL1 gene, in 2001 (Pray, 2008). Yet, product approvals are non-existent for more than 95% of rare diseases (Kaufmann et al., 2018), frequently necessitating decades-old ther-apeutic paradigms that appear more suitable for a discussion of history, not modern science. Huntington's disease serves as a sobering example. When George Huntington, recently graduated from Columbia Medical School, published in 1872 (Huntington, 1872) on the disease eventually named after him, it generated more interest, even in his day, than afforded most rare diseases. He was in touch with some eminent clinicians of the day and expressed hope that science would one day provide answers; yet, 150 years after Huntington's seminal account, while the genetic cause has been isolated, and medications can reduce choreic movement and ease psy-chiatric symptoms, the treatment summary provided online by the Mayo Clinic begins with a blunt assessment, "No treatments can alter the course of Huntington's disease" (Mayo Clinic, 2020). Over the past century and a half, the circumstances have changed yet fundamentally stayed the same.

1.2 Definitions

The notion of rare disease has been defined variously across geographies. Perhaps most cited is from the Orphan Drug Act passed by the US con-gress in 1983, leading the Food and Drug Administration (FDA) to label a disease as rare if it affects fewer than 200,000 people in the United States (FDA, 2020). In the European Union, as stated by the European Medicines Agency, a disease is defined as rare if it affects fewer than five in 10,000 people across the European Union (European Medicines Agency, 2018). In Japan, according to the Ministry of Health, Labour and Welfare, such dis-eases are defined as those affecting fewer than 50,000 people, or one in 2,500 people (Hayashi and Umeda, 2008; Ministry of Health, Labour and Welfare, 2009). Globally, the World Health Organization uses a prevalence of 0.065%–0.1%. It is commonly estimated that around 10% of the global population suffers from a rare disease, with around 250 new such diseases identified each year (Dawkins et al., 2018), although these obviously vary by the definition applied. Hence, while being individually rare, the cur-rently identified rare diseases are collectively not rare at the population level (Griggs et al., 2009).

1.3 Differences in Clinical Setting for Rare Diseases

As development of therapies inevitably follows clinical understanding, we should first consider a few differences in the clinical understanding of rare diseases.

1.3.1 Understanding of the Disease

Clinical understanding of the disease can frequently be uncertain, and it is possible that little to no research has been conducted previously, especially in disease subtypes. The underlying cause of the disease may or may not be known. Treatment guidance documents may be out of date or non-existent (Stoller, 2018). Identification of key prognostic factors may be difficult to identify yet particularly important to incorporate into the design (e.g. as stratification factors) of small studies, which are prone to imbalance and bias. The number of clinicians (and hence program development leads) with experience in the area will likely be limited, prompting more "on-the-job" learning for the development team. How best to measure disease progression or remission may also be unclear, which creates uncertainty as to the best endpoints to use in a clinical trial. FDA guidance on rare disease drug development (FDA, 2019) indicates that "For many rare diseases, well-characterized efficacy endpoints appropriate for the disease are not available."

1.3.2 Identification and Diagnosis of Patients

Patients with rare diseases often endure years of symptoms before gaining a diagnosis. In the case of children, the average is 6–8 years before a diagnosis is obtained (World Economic Forum, 2020). Over 40% of patients obtain an incorrect diagnosis more than once. As a result, the patients can be difficult to identify, particularly in commercial databases, such as insurance claims databases. Also, the patients can finally present at study screening in widely varying states of disease. A 2019 survey from Tufts University (Burton et al., 2021; Tufts Center for the Study of Drug Development, 2019) found that approximately 81% of screened patients were ineligible to enroll and 56% failed to be randomized in rare disease clinical trials, versus 57% and 36% of patients who fell into the categories in non-rare disease trials. Even once identified and enrolled, retention may suffer if desperate patients discontinue to try other, even off-label, therapies.

1.3.3 Funding Challenges

It only makes sense that a disease which has fewer patients will have a lower potential for revenues. As a result, many rare disease researchers struggle at the outset to obtain funding in pursuit of therapies. To compensate, the standards for clinical benefit (and price) may need to be altered to justify the up-front investment risk.

For fiscal year 2019, the National Institutes of Health was appropriated $39 billion, of which only $38 million (0.1%) was awarded to study a wide range of rare diseases (Zhu et al., 2021). However, there have been efforts to increase funding for rare diseases. In October of 2021, the FDA announced 11 new congressionally funded clinical trial research grants, awarded by FDA's Orphan Products Grants Program, which sums to more than $25 million of funding for rare diseases over 4 years (FDA, 2021).

1.3.4 Regulatory Uncertainties

A lack of clear precedents, as is usually the case, can leave sponsors uncertain how any particular development scenarios or choices will be received. Standards, such as orphan drug designation (discussed in a later chapter), have been developed to aid in this understanding, but considerable risk and uncertainty remain. This uncertainty extends to the payor domain, often critical in rare diseases in which the patients can generally not be expected to afford cutting-edge therapies on their own. As a result, studies specifically targeting payor requirements across varying geographies may be needed.

1.3.5 Privacy Considerations

Clearly, avoiding identification of specific patients is a greater challenge when there are fewer patients with the condition. As a result, following privacy regulations and reporting practices that reduce this possibility is important in the rare disease space. For example, reporting patients with a specific rare genotype might constitute a small enough group to allow identification based on other information (e.g. country, age, and gender). Generally, no groups smaller than a pre-specified size (e.g. 5) are reported.

1.3.6 Pediatric Focus

Approximately 80% of rare diseases are inherited, and most of those patients are children (Wright et al., 2018). This fact touches on many of the development aspects already mentioned. Recruitment activities (including informed consent) are more complicated due to the need to involve parents/guardians; data collection for some endpoints, such as subjective patient-reported outcomes, may be even less certain; and additional privacy/transparency requirements may apply. Recruitment of pediatric patients in pre-market studies is more widely conducted than in common diseases, which often only enroll patients once a therapy is marketed.

1.4 Scope

In the remainder of this work, we will attempt to give an overview of the clinical development implications of researching new therapies in this area.

The emphasis is on scientific and, in particular, clinical data-driven considerations, and not on issues which are purely operational, manufacturing, legal, or commercial in nature. (While basic research and non-clinical studies are critical to the development of any new therapy and may differ in nature for rare diseases, they are not in the already wide scope we attempt to purview. Neither are the legal/regulatory ramifications associated with privacy concerns.) However, these quantitative issues are addressed in a non-technical way with most technical statistical considerations left to references provided. After some discussion of the developmental implications of the rare disease setting, we will provide clinical case studies of approaches increasingly leveraged therein. We will also provide a summary of the various regulatory designations and options which figure more prominently for rare diseases. A chapter on modeling and simulation approaches to bridge notable data gaps is presented, followed by another approach for additional relevant information, real-world evidence. Last, we look at how these elements come together for the prototypical rare disease patient: the child (Wright et al., 2018). These works are written with the general clinical research audience in mind, hopeful that the collected works herein can shed light on both the rewarding opportunities and the undeniable challenges which coexist in clinical research for rare diseases.

References

Burton, A., Castaño, A., Bruno, M., Riley, S., Schumacher, J., Sultan, M. B., Tai, S. S., Judge, D. P., Patel, J. K., & Kelly, J. W. (2021). Drug Discovery and Development in Rare Diseases: Taking a Closer Look at the Tafamidis Story. *Drug Design, Development and Therapy*, *15*, 1225–1243. https://doi.org/10.2147/DDDT. S289772

Dawkins, H. J. S., Draghia-Akli, R., Lasko, P., Lau, L. P. L., Jonker, A. H., Cutillo, C. M., Rath, A., Boycott, K. M., Baynam, G., Lochmüller, H., Kaufmann, P., Le Cam, Y., Hivert, V., Austin, C. P., & Consortium (IRDiRC), I. R. D. R. (2018). Progress in Rare Diseases Research 2010–2016: An IRDiRC Perspective. *Clinical and Translational Science*, *11*(1), 11–20. https://doi.org/10.1111/cts.12501

EMA. (2018). *Committee for Orphan Medicinal Products (COMP)*. European Medicines Agency. https://www.ema.europa.eu/en/committees/committee-orphan-medicinal-products-comp

FDA. (2019). *Rare Diseases: Common Issues in Drug Development Guidance for Industry*. https://www.fda.gov/regulatory-information/search-fda-guidance-documents/rare-diseases-common-issues-drug-development-guidance-industry

FDA. (2020). *Rare Diseases at FDA*. https://www.fda.gov/patients/rare-diseases-fda

FDA. (2021). *FDA Awards 11 Grants to Clinical Trials to Develop New Medical Products for Rare Disease Treatments*. https://www.fda.gov/news-events/press-announcements/fda-awards-11-grants-clinical-trials-develop-new-medical-products-rare-disease-treatments

Griggs, R. C., Batshaw, M., Dunkle, M., Gopal-Srivastava, R., Kaye, E., Krischer, J., Nguyen, T., Paulus, K., & Merkel, P. A. (2009). Clinical Research for Rare Disease: Opportunities, Challenges, and Solutions. *Molecular Genetics and Metabolism, 96*(1), 20–26. https://doi.org/10.1016/j.ymgme.2008.10.003

Haendel, M., Vasilevsky, N., Unni, D., Bologa, C., Harris, N., Rehm, H., Hamosh, A., Baynam, G., Groza, T., McMurry, J., Dawkins, H., Rath, A., Thaxon, C., Bocci, G., Joachimiak, M. P., Köhler, S., Robinson, P. N., Mungall, C., & Oprea, T. I. (2020). How Many Rare Diseases Are There? *Nature Reviews Drug Discovery, 19*(2), 77–78. https://doi.org/10.1038/d41573-019-00180-y

Hayashi, S., & Umeda, T. (2008). 35 Years of Japanese Policy on Rare Diseases. *The Lancet, 372*(9642), 889–890. https://doi.org/10.1016/S0140-6736(08)61393-8

Huntington, G. (1872). On Chorea. *Medical and Surgical Reporter of Philadelphia, 26*(15), 317–321.

Kaufmann, P., Pariser, A. R., & Austin, C. (2018). From Scientific Discovery to Treatments for Rare Diseases – The View from the National Center for Advancing Translational Sciences – Office of Rare Diseases Research. *Orphanet Journal of Rare Diseases, 13*(1), 196. https://doi.org/10.1186/s13023-018-0936-x

Mayo Clinic. (2020). *Huntington's Disease—Diagnosis and Treatment.* https://www.mayoclinic.org/diseases-conditions/huntingtons-disease/diagnosis-treatment/drc-20356122

MHLW. (2009). *Overview of Orphan Drug/Medical Device Designation System.* https://www.mhlw.go.jp/english/policy/health-medical/pharmaceuticals/orphan_drug.html

Miller, K. L., Fermaglich, L. J., & Maynard, J. (2021). Using Four Decades of FDA Orphan Drug Designations to Describe Trends in Rare Disease Drug Development: Substantial Growth Seen in Development of Drugs for Rare Oncologic, Neurologic, and Pediatric-Onset Diseases. *Orphanet Journal of Rare Diseases, 16*(1), 265. https://doi.org/10.1186/s13023-021-01901-6

NIH. (2020). *Rare Diseases.* https://www.nih.gov/about-nih/what-we-do/nih-turning-discovery-into-health/rare-diseases

Pray, L. (2008). Gleevec: The Breakthrough in Cancer Treatment. *Nature Education, 1*(1), 37.

Stoller, J. K. (2018). The Challenge of Rare Diseases. *Chest, 153*(6), 1309–1314. https://doi.org/10.1016/j.chest.2017.12.018

Tufts Center for the Study of Drug Development. (2019). *Growth in Rare Disease R&D is Challenging Development Strategy and Execution.* Tufts University.

World Economic Forum. (2020). *It Takes Far Too Long for a Rare Disease to be Diagnosed. Here's how that can Change.* https://www.weforum.org/agenda/2020/02/it-takes-far-too-long-for-a-rare-disease-to-be-diagnosed-heres-how-that-can-change/

Wright, C. F., FitzPatrick, D. R., & Firth, H. V. (2018). Paediatric Genomics: Diagnosing Rare Disease in Children. *Nature Reviews Genetics, 19*(5), 253–268. https://doi.org/10.1038/nrg.2017.116

Zhu, Q., Nguyên, Đ.-T., Sheils, T., Alyea, G., Sid, E., Xu, Y., Dickens, J., Mathé, E. A., & Pariser, A. (2021). Scientific Evidence Based Rare Disease Research Discovery with Research Funding Data in Knowledge Graph. *Orphanet Journal of Rare Diseases, 16*, 483. https://doi.org/10.1186/s13023-021-02120-9

2

Challenges and Opportunities in Rare Disease Drug Development

Glen Laird

Vertex Pharmaceuticals

CONTENTS

2.1 Introduction

Development strategies pursued by sponsors are often directly related to the context of the clinical, scientific, and regulatory environment presented by the disease. Several aspects regarding rare diseases have a direct implication on the clinical development of novel therapies. In the case of rare diseases, an efficient development path is often both necessary and possible to pursue. Typically, there is a high unmet medical need presented by a serious disease. Also, the small number of patients can obviously limit study sample size. Both the EMA and FDA (EMA, 2006; FDA, 2019c) have published guidance to discuss these issues and what sponsors should consider to addressing these issues in drug development for small populations/rare diseases. The FDA guidance notes that

> Although the statutory requirements for marketing approval for drugs to treat rare and common diseases are the same and issues ... are encountered in other drug development programs, these issues are frequently more difficult to address in the context of a rare disease for which there is often limited medical and scientific knowledge, natural history data, and drug development experience.

DOI: 10.1201/9781003080954-2

These and other factors combine to create certain development trends, including focused recruitment efforts, the use of innovative study designs, incorporation of external data, biomarkers, integration of modeling and simulation (M&S), expanded regulatory pathways, and the desire for transformative therapies.

2.2 Focused Recruitment Efforts

Much discussion of rare diseases must begin with the simple fact that it can be difficult to enroll patients when very few exist. The patients who do exist may be difficult to identify, especially in large, broad databases. Diagnoses for these patients are commonly wrong and/or belated (National Organization for Rare Disorders, 2020). As a result, recruitment may often need to take place at specialized clinics which understand the disease and treat the correct patients frequently. Patient advocacy organizations may also play a role in patient identification and characterization (Stoller, 2018). A "feeder study" simply to identify patients in the population can be considered if a particular mutation or subtype of disease is desired for study which may be difficult to enroll. Such identified patients could then quickly be enrolled in a future interventional study without delay. If the geography of the available patients is wide, a decentralized, or even fully remote study could be considered in which patient visits to enrolling site are minimal to none (Van Norman, 2021). Even if a focused recruitment approach is possible, practicality may require actual inclusion criteria for rare disease clinical trials be broader than those used for trials of common diseases (FDA, 2019c). In that case, pre-specified considerations and analyses for the breadth of subpopulations therein (e.g. subgroup analyses, weighted estimates, sensitivity analyses, and covariate adjustment) can be important for rigor and generalizability. The size of the safety database may be one of the practical considerations.

It is worth noting that rare disease studies often need analogously focused retention efforts (Augustine et al., 2013). Most patients in these studies do not have the luxury of participating in a study "for the good of science." Specific therapeutic or financial benefits generally need to be maintained throughout the course of the study to avoid patient dropout (Stoller, 2018). For example, a short period of potentially receiving placebo treatment may be acceptable in some contexts, but only if it is known to be followed by an extended treatment period on therapy expected to be effective. Since many genetic diseases are lifelong, involving a gradual clinical decline, long-term data are often key to a complete benefit–risk picture, making efforts to avoid of dropout/missing data even more important.

2.3 Use of Innovative Study Designs and Analyses

The use of study designs beyond the traditional designs is common and even necessary due to limitations in sample size and prior information, as well as unmet clinical need. Randomized, blinded, parallel group, placebo-controlled studies standard in many disease areas may be impractical, inefficient, or even unethical in the rare disease setting. A subsequent chapter will present case studies on a "basket study," in which several potential subtypes of disease are studied simultaneously. There is also a chapter highlighting several trial design and analysis options that may have particular appeal in the rare disease setting. These include sample size re-estimation, exact group sequential designs, and phase 2/3 treatment selection designs. (In this context, "treatment selection" may include selection from several doses or regimens of the same therapy.) According to the book by Chow (2020), the FDA's guidance on adaptive designs (FDA, 2019a) indicates that "adaptive seamless trial designs may allow early evidence to be used later in a study, especially helpful when there are limited numbers of patients to study." In addition, the same guidance also implies that "key features of the trial design and preplanned analyses should be discussed with the review division before trial initiation." From an analysis perspective, a simulated-supported overview of multiple endpoints analyses is also summarized in the same chapter of the current work. Approaches detailed in prior works include dose–response (FDA, 2003; ICH-E4, 1994), randomized withdrawal (FDA, 2019b), and randomized start/delayed start (D'Agostino, 2009; Spineli et al., 2017) designs. In common, these approaches attempt to efficiently use all available information in the demonstration of efficacy. Exposing only the minimum needed number of patients to placebo (or therapies not expected to be sufficiently effective) is often paramount. A greater proportion of patients on the registrational dose (or a higher dose) also allows for a safety database more likely to be viewed as sufficient in a small study. (While ICH E1A (FDA, 1995) mentions that a smaller number of patients may be acceptable for safety assessment when the intended treatment population is small, sufficient exposure for adequate safety evaluation is still needed.)

2.4 Use of Data External to Clinical Trials

In some cases, data external to a clinical trial may be used to fill in gaps related to a limited understanding of the disease, such disease prevalence or how correlated various outcomes are with particular clinical measurements. In some cases, past clinical trials can be used. Increasingly, however, alternative data sources are leveraged, especially for rare diseases, which typically have few prior clinical studies. A subsequent chapter specifically deals with the use of real-world evidence (RWE) in support of drug development. RWE, evidence derived from real-world data, has various definitions around the regulatory landscape, but common examples of real-world data include electronic health records, insurance claims databases, and patient registries. FDA guidance on the use of RWE was published in December 2021 (FDA, 2021a), which emphasized the need to employ reliable fit for purpose data, pre-specification of key analyses, and early engagement with the agency. Chapter 6 will discuss the use of RWE in the rare disease setting.

A particular version of incorporating information external to a clinical trial is the use of a natural history study (NHS), in which patients are followed, usually longitudinally, on the course of their disease, generally when no effective therapy is available. To date, data collection has usually been retrospective, rather than prospective, for operational reasons, although a prospective design has scientific advantages (Jahanshahi et al., 2021). FDA discussion on an NHS was included in guidance for rare disease populations (FDA, 2019c). It notes that an NHS is not required but may provide additional disease understanding and, in special circumstances (unmet need, predictable disease, and large drug effect temporally associated with the therapy), can provide an external control group for interventional trials. Availability and consistency of important prognostic covariates can be a key issue with historical data, including NHS. Case studies using electronic health records and NHSs are presented in later chapters.

2.5 Strong Incorporation of Biomarkers

There are two major dimensions to the incorporation of biomarkers. As many rare diseases have specific genetic etiologies, population (or subpopulation) selection is a natural employment of biomarkers in rare disease clinical trials. Non-standard upfront genetic testing may be required to verify the patient is in the group of interest. Frequently, these are patients with more severe manifestations of a disease. When multiple disease subtypes are involved in a study, biomarkers often serve as the dividing line for those subtypes. The FDA guidance on rare diseases (FDA, 2019c) highlights the importance of sensitivity (true-positive rate), specificity (true-negative rate), range of measurement, and reproducibility of any biomarker assay. Sometimes, complex series of analyses can be involved related to multiple subtypes defined by biomarkers.

As long-term clinical outcomes can frequently be difficult to observe in a feasible timeframe for all patients, especially if a small population size leads to low enrollment rates, the other major dimension to the use of a subset of biomarkers is as surrogate endpoints. The guidance for industry and FDA staff Qualification Process for Drug Development Tools (FDA, 2020) includes important information about the features of biomarkers used as endpoints. Various definitions of surrogate endpoints exist in the literature, but broadly speaking, a surrogate endpoint is a substitute, generally intermediate, endpoint that may reasonably be expected to predict patient benefit. Many clinical studies across a wide array of therapeutic areas include biomarker endpoints. However, for many of those areas, biomarker endpoints are treated as strictly exploratory in nature, with few having an ultimate impact on the success of the study, especially from a regulatory perspective. Typically, "extensive evidence must accumulate, including evidence from epidemiological and clinical trials" (FDA, 2018) for such an endpoint to be acceptable as a surrogate endpoint. As a result, their overall use as secondary or even primary endpoints is uncommon. However, in rare disease studies, the use of biomarker endpoints as primary or secondary endpoints is more frequent and warrants careful considerations (Kakkis et al., 2015). The FDA maintains a list of currently accepted surrogate endpoints (FDA, 2022b), which contains endpoints for a number of rare diseases. However, a biomarker endpoint not included in the current list is not automatically disqualified from consideration as a registrational endpoint depending on the specifics of a given study and disease. A subsequent chapter gives a case study in the use of a surrogate endpoint for registration of a Duchenne muscular dystrophy therapy.

Diseases affecting muscular movement also provide an example of another category of surrogate endpoint: digital health technologies, such as wearable accelerometers, employed in some studies of Parkinson's disease allow for near-constant measurement of movements over a longer period, and these devices have potential to mitigate both the challenge of sample size, via collection of additional data per subject, reducing variability, and the challenge of poor disease area knowledge, via allowing greater choices for endpoint definitions and timing. In this regard, for a rare disease with limited prior study, predicting in what exact fashion a treatment effect may be detectable is difficult; having longitudinal data across several dimensions can be advantageous. Not surprisingly, they also involve challenges to understand the multiplicity-driven type 1 error (false-positive rate) inflation that can accompany such a range of choices, as well as missing data issues arising from non-compliance, battery failure, poor device placement, or other operational obstacles. For Duchenne muscular dystrophy, the EMA has issued a qualification opinion on the use of 95th percentile of stride velocity as an acceptable secondary endpoint in pivotal or exploratory drug therapeutic studies for regulatory purposes when measured by a "valid and suitable wearable device" (EMA, 2019). Muscular disease is only one relatively advanced example as digital health technologies are being investigated more broadly in other areas (e.g. cough, heart rate, and pain) and have warranted issuance of FDA Guidance (FDA, 2021b).

2.6 M&S Input to Development Choices

Information gaps presented by the rare disease setting can potentially be mitigated by various approaches. In addition to the use of efficient clinical study designs, the use of M&S approaches may also be employed in the name of efficiency. The discipline of pharmacometrics and its implementation in model informed drug development are described in a subsequent chapter. Frequently, pharmacometrics models use a full time series of patient data (e.g. pharmacokinetic and pharmacodynamic data) to inform key development decisions such as dose selection and extrapolation to additional populations, such as children or vulnerable patient populations. Pediatric extrapolation is also discussed in a subsequent chapter on pediatric clinical development for rare diseases. Bayesian approaches to modeling are also outlined in that chapter. Value added from M&S may go hand in hand with the use of biomarkers to capture key concepts.

2.7 Expanded Regulatory Options

As previously alluded, the clinical context of many rare diseases provides a setting for regulatory options not as frequently attainable in more common therapeutic areas. One of these, orphan drug designation, is explicitly reserved for rare indications. Orphan drug designation has somewhat different flavors in the United States and Europe, but both offer incentives (e.g. protocol assistance, market exclusivity, and fee reductions) for development in rare diseases. The serious nature of many rare diseases also affords additional regulatory options. Tools such as breakthrough designation, accelerated approval, or regenerative medicine advanced therapy are not reserved for rare diseases but are frequently used therein. Additional incentives exist related to pediatric development. Without these various regulatory options, the limited number of patients may make novel therapies impractical from both a development and market perspective. While not an avowedly rare disease vehicle, the FDA pilot program for complex innovative designs (CID) (FDA, 2022a) may provide additional FDA feedback for complex designs, often involving detailed simulations, which may organically arise from the rare disease setting. A summary of the programs accepted thus far, including some with small populations, is available from Price and Scott (2021).

2.8 The Desire for Transformative Therapies

The challenges awaiting sponsors weighing clinical development in a rare disease are considerable and somewhat particular to the space. These challenges often create a focus on transformative therapies as modest improvements may not be viable to overcome the limitations imposed from both a development (e.g. study sample size) and commercial (e.g. reimbursement agreements) point of view. The ascertainment of a minimally clinically important difference is often not sufficiently explored (or agreed upon) in a rare disease population, so an incontrovertible treatment effect target can be clarifying, particularly in settings that do not involve randomized comparisons.

The challenges for development in rare diseases are certainly substantial. However, the promise of a decisive accomplishment is also substantial. Successful navigation of the challenges faced can not only dramatically improve the lives of patients desperately waiting at the curb of the innovation highway but also pave the way to future successes heretofore hidden around the corner.

References

Augustine, E. F., Adams, H. R., & Mink, J. W. (2013). Clinical Trials in Rare Disease: Challenges and Opportunities. *Journal of Child Neurology, 28*(9), 1142–1150. https://doi.org/10.1177/0883073813495959

Chow, S.-C. (2020). *Innovative Methods for Rare Disease Drug Development*. Chapman and Hall/CRC. Boca Raton, FL.

D'Agostino, R. B. (2009). The Delayed-Start Study Design. *New England Journal of Medicine, 361*(13), 1304–1306. https://doi.org/10.1056/NEJMsm0904209

EMA. (2006). *Guideline on Clinical Trials in Small Populations*. https://www.ema.europa.eu/en/documents/scientific-guideline/guideline-clinical-trials-small-populations_en.pdf

EMA. (2019). *Qualification Opinion on Stride Velocity 95th Centile as a Secondary Endpoint in Duchenne Muscular Dystrophy Measured by a Valid and Suitable Wearable Device**. https://www.ema.europa.eu/en/documents/scientific-guideline/qualification-opinion-stride-velocity-95th-centile-secondary-endpoint-duchenne-muscular-dystrophy_en.pdf

FDA. (1995). *E1A The Extent of Population Exposure to Assess Clinical Safety: For Drugs Intended for Long-term Treatment of Non-Life-Threatening Conditions*. U.S. Food and Drug Administration. https://www.fda.gov/regulatory-information/search-fda-guidance-documents/e1a-extent-population-exposure-assess-clinical-safety-drugs-intended-long-term-treatment-non-life

FDA. (2003). *Exposure-Response Relationships—Study Design, Data Analysis, and Regulatory Applications*. https://www.fda.gov/regulatory-information/search-fda-guidance-documents/exposure-response-relationships-study-design-data-analysis-and-regulatory-applications

FDA. (2018). *Surrogate Endpoint Resources for Drug and Biologic Development*. FDA. https://www.fda.gov/drugs/development-resources/surrogate-endpoint-resources-drug-and-biologic-development

FDA. (2019a). Adoptive Design Clinical Trails for Drugs and Bilogics Guidance for Industry. U.S. Food and Drug Administration. https://www.fda.gov/regulatory-information/search-fda-guidance-documents/adaptive-design-clinical-trials-drugs-and-biologics-guidance-industry

FDA. (2019b). *Enrichment Strategies for Clinical Trials to Support Approval of Human Drugs and Biological Products*. https://www.fda.gov/regulatory-information/search-fda-guidance-documents/enrichment-strategies-clinical-trials-support-approval-human-drugs-and-biological-products

FDA. (2019c). *Rare Diseases: Common Issues in Drug Development Guidance for Industry*. https://www.fda.gov/regulatory-information/search-fda-guidance-documents/rare-diseases-common-issues-drug-development-guidance-industry

FDA. (2020). *Qualification Process for Drug Development Tools Guidance for Industry and FDA Staff*. https://www.fda.gov/regulatory-information/search-fda-guidance-documents/qualification-process-drug-development-tools-guidance-industry-and-fda-staff

FDA. (2021a). *Considerations for the Use of Real-World Data and Real-World Evidence to Support Regulatory Decision-Making for Drug and Biological Products*. https://www.fda.gov/regulatory-information/search-fda-guidance-documents/considerations-use-real-world-data-and-real-world-evidence-support-regulatory-decision-making-drug

FDA. (2021b). *Digital Health Technologies for Remote Data Acquisition in Clinical Investigations*. https://www.fda.gov/regulatory-information/search-fda-guidance-documents/digital-health-technologies-remote-data-acquisition-clinical-investigations

FDA. (2022a). *Complex innovative Trial Design Pilot Meeting Program*. https://www.fda.gov/drugs/development-resources/complex-innovative-trial-design-pilot-meeting-program

FDA. (2022b). *Table of Surrogate Endpoints That Were the Basis of Drug Approval or Licensure*. https://www.fda.gov/drugs/development-resources/table-surrogate-endpoints-were-basis-drug-approval-or-licensure

ICH-E4. (1994). *E4 Dose-Response Information to Support Drug Registration*. https://www.fda.gov/media/71279/download

Jahanshahi, M., Gregg, K., Davis, G., Ndu, A., Miller, V., Vockley, J., Ollivier, C., Franolic, T., & Sakai, S. (2021). The Use of External Controls in FDA Regulatory Decision Making. *Therapeutic Innovation & Regulatory Science, 55*(5), 1019–1035. https://doi.org/10.1007/s43441-021-00302-y

Kakkis, E. D., O'Donovan, M., Cox, G., Hayes, M., Goodsaid, F., Tandon, P., Furlong, P., Boynton, S., Bozic, M., Orfali, M., & Thornton, M. (2015). Recommendations for the Development of Rare Disease Drugs Using the Accelerated Approval Pathway and for Qualifying Biomarkers as Primary Endpoints. *Orphanet Journal of Rare Diseases, 10*, 16. https://doi.org/10.1186/s13023-014-0195-4

National Organization for Rare Disorders (NORD). (2020). *Barriers to Rare Disease Diagnosis, Care, and Treatment in the US: A 30-year Comparative Analysis*. https://rarediseases.org/wp-content/uploads/2020/11/NRD-2088-Barriers-30-Yr-Survey-Report_FNL-2.pdf

Price, D., & Scott, J. (2021). The U.S. Food and Drug Administration's Complex Innovative Trial Design Pilot Meeting Program: Progress to date. *Clinical Trials, 18*(6), 706–710. https://doi.org/10.1177/17407745211050580

Spineli, L. M., Jenz, E., Großhennig, A., & Koch, A. (2017). Critical Appraisal of Arguments for the Delayed-Start Design Proposed as Alternative to the Parallel-Group Randomized Clinical Trial Design in the Field of Rare Disease. *Orphanet Journal of Rare Diseases, 12*, 140. https://doi.org/10.1186/s13023-017-0692-3

Stoller, J. K. (2018). The Challenge of Rare Diseases. *Chest, 153*(6), 1309–1314. https://doi.org/10.1016/j.chest.2017.12.018

Van Norman, G. A. (2021). Decentralized Clinical Trials. *JACC: Basic to Translational Science, 6*(4), 384–387. https://doi.org/10.1016/j.jacbts.2021.01.011.

3

Developing Drugs for Rare Diseases: Regulatory Strategies and Considerations

Joanne Palmisano

Vertex Pharmaceuticals, Retired

CONTENTS

DOI: 10.1201/9781003080954-3

3.1 Introduction

Advances in pharmaceutical science and biotechnology, including advances in cellular and gene product development, have contributed to a global acceleration in the number of novel medicinal products in development aimed at addressing serious unmet medical needs in rare and orphan disease. Given the unique and often small patient populations associated with these conditions, regulatory health authorities have established guidelines that govern orphan and rare disease drug development, which can differ across global regions. In this chapter, the term *drug* will refer to all therapeutic modalities, such as small molecules, biologics, cellular and genetic therapies, and drug-device or drug-biologic combinations. Similarly, the mention of *the drug development program* refers to the inclusive requirements for nonclinical, clinical, and product manufacturing elements of the program.

This chapter will focus on established regulatory pathways of the US Food and Drug Administration (FDA) and the European Union (EU) European Medicines Agency (EMA), which represent the major health authorities governing rare and orphan disease drug development. This is not to dismiss the consideration of other regional health authorities, including Japan PMDA/MHLW, Health Canada, UK MHRA, Swissmedic, Brazil's ANVISA, and Australia's TGA, among others. As drug development for rare disease is increasingly global and multiregional, it is important to give attention to regional health authority requirements necessary for the registration and marketing of drugs where the intended patient populations are served. Early discussions with regional health authorities and health technology assessment (HTA) bodies for agreement on the required elements of the proposed nonclinical, clinical, and product manufacturing development and marketing plans for a novel treatment are recommended.

In general, the same expectations and considerations for the development of medicines for human use for any disease or condition also apply for rare and orphan diseases. The International Council for Harmonisation of Technical Requirements for Pharmaceuticals for Human Use (ICH) has established guidelines that are accepted by global regulatory authorities and industry partners outlining the scientific and technical aspects of human drug development. The goal of these mutually developed guidelines is "to achieve greater harmonisation worldwide to ensure that safe, effective and high quality medicines are developed, and registered and maintained in the most resource efficient manner whilst meeting high standards." The ICH website (https://www.ich.org/) provides information and training materials on all current and planned guidelines.

What is unique to rare and orphan disease is the mutual urgency of sponsors and regulators to respond to the high unmet need of patients with these disorders who have none or few satisfactory therapeutic options for treatment. This has resulted in regulatory pathways for the acceleration of development of new medicines and programs that expedite the review of these applications in support of early access for patients.

In the development of priority medicines, an important consideration has been placed by the FDA and EMA regarding the challenges for sponsors to complete quality and manufacturing development, including data requirements for such, in conjunction with accelerated clinical development in expedited programs (Breakthrough Therapy Designation (BTD), Regenerative Medicine Advanced Therapy (RMAT), PRIority MEdicines (PRIME)) in time for approval/marketing authorization. The regulatory requirements for chemistry, manufacturing, and control, and the quality requirements for advanced medicinal products (cellular and genetic therapies) are beyond the scope of this chapter. The reader is referred to available FDA and EMA guidance to support quality development in early access programs that reflect the effort for alignment of both agencies to adopt common regulatory approaches, given the global nature of drug development. Early engagement with regulators for quality and manufacturing topics is encouraged to be in parallel with regulatory consultations on the nonclinical and clinical development programs.

For a comprehensive overview of all published regional guidance for the development of human medicines including regulatory programs and procedures, refer to the websites of the FDA (www.fda.gov) and the EMA (www.ema.europa.eu). Other regional regulatory authority requirements likewise can be accessed via their websites, for example, Health Canada (https://www.canada.ca/en/health-canada.html) and Japan's PMDA/MHLW (https://www.pmda.go.jp/english/).

3.2 Expedited Programs and Accelerated Review Pathways of the US FDA

The US FDA has introduced into the Code of Federal Regulations both procedural and statutory approaches to support expedited drug development and the review and approval process for drugs for serious or life-threatening conditions, with the intention to accelerating access to new medicines addressing the high unmet medical need [*Drugs Intended to Treat Life-Threatening and Severely-Debilitating Illnesses. 21 CFR §312.80* (2020) https://www.ecfr.gov/current/title-21]. While the statutory standards of safety and effectiveness apply to all drug approvals, the purpose of this code has determined that it is appropriate for the US FDA to apply

> the broadest flexibility in applying the statutory standards, while preserving appropriate guarantees for safety and effectiveness... in recognition that physicians and patients are generally willing to accept

greater risks or side effects from products that treat life-threatening and severely-debilitating illnesses, than they would accept from products that treat less serious illnesses.

These programs and pathways, which include the orphan drug designation (ODD) (1983), fast track (FT) (1988), the accelerated approval (AA) pathway (1992), priority review (PR) (1992), breakthrough therapy designation (2012), and regenerative medicine advanced therapy designation (2016), are designed to assist sponsors in working with the FDA to expedite the development, review, and approval of such medicines. Guidance documents that describe the US FDA thinking and requirements for these programs can be accessed at [https://www.fda.gov/regulatory-information/search-fda-guidance-documents/] and are captured in FDA Guidance for Industry-Expedited Programs for Serious Conditions, Drugs and Biologics (May 2014) and in Expedited Programs for Regenerative Medicine Therapies for Serious Conditions (February 2019).

Although these programs offer different opportunities for expediting drug development, there is a good deal of overlap between them. Sponsors may apply for and receive more than one designation for a given product, but applications are separate, and the same supporting information can be utilized. Early engagement with the designated division of the FDA is expected to establish the intent for expedited development and gain regulatory guidance on the required elements for the development program and future application to support the statutory requirements for the demonstration of product efficacy and safety in the intended population.

In the regulations and guidance adopted for access to these programs, the FDA defines a serious or life-threatening disease or condition as that which impacts survival and/or day-to-day function such that if left untreated, it will progress from a less severe condition to a more serious one. The FDA evaluates the applications for these programs based on similar criteria for the potential of the drug to meet one or more of the following criteria:

- The potential to demonstrate improved effectiveness on outcomes for a serious condition
- The potential to avoid serious side effects of an available therapy
- The potential to improve the diagnosis of a serious condition where early diagnosis results in an improved outcome
- The potential to decrease a clinically significant toxicity of an available therapy that is common and causes discontinuation of treatment
- The potential to have the ability to address emerging or anticipated public health need.

3.2.1 US FDA Orphan Drug Designation (ODD)

The Orphan Drug Act of 1983 established the definition of an orphan (rare) disease as

> any disease or condition which occurs so infrequently in the U.S. that there is no reasonable expectation that the cost of developing and making available in the United States a drug for such disease or condition will be recovered from sales in the United States of such drug.

In 1984, the ODA was amended, redefining rare diseases as those affecting less than 200,000 persons in the United States or, for a vaccine, diagnostic drug, or preventive drug to be administered to 200,000 or more persons per year, where the drug will not be profitable within 7 years following FDA approval. This US law is important as it led to the establishment of the Office of Orphan Products Development, which oversees the provisions for incentives to make development of drugs intended to treat small populations financially viable, especially for small pharmaceutical or biotechnology companies or academic researchers with limited resources to transform a potential novel drug candidate into a marketed product.

The ODA established a pathway for a promising new therapy to receive an orphan designation (OD) status based on preliminary data providing evidence for an expectation of favorable efficacy in the intended serious condition. The scientific rationale, including in vitro, in vivo, and/or clinical study data if available, in support of the expectation that the drug has promise to treat, diagnose, or prevent the disease or condition is provided in the application for orphan designation.

The receipt of orphan drug status grants provisional entitlement to the financial incentives available under the act, including tax credits for clinical trial costs, fee exemptions at the time of marketing application, and eligibility of 7-year market exclusivity, should the drug successfully secure marketing approval from the FDA. If the drug is similar to a previously approved drug, the demonstration of clinical superiority at the time of approval is required. Applications for OD designation are submitted to the Office of Orphan Products Development and evaluated according to the merits of the application within 60 days. Once the OD status is achieved, the application moves to the relevant review division within the FDA, either in the Center for Drug Evaluation and Research Office of New Drugs for drug and biological therapeutics or in the Center for Biologics Evaluation and Research (CBER) for biological products derived from human blood, stem cells or tissue, genetic therapies, and vaccines [https://www.fda.gov/industry/developing-products-rare-diseases-conditions/designating-orphan-product-drugs-and-biological-products].

The OD designation alone does not confer on the sponsor the ability to start clinical development of a new drug. The sponsor must first submit an Investigational New Drug (IND) application to the designated FDA division for review and approval to begin the clinical testing in humans. US requirements for conducting research in human subjects are based on shared ethical principles and are consistent with internationally recognized ethical standards intended to ensure the rights and safety of human subjects in clinical trials. These standards are described in the Declaration of Helsinki [https://www.wma.net/policies-post/wma-declaration-of-helsinki-ethical-principles-for-medical-research-involving-human-subjects/] and have been codified in US law in the Code of Federal Regulations Title 21 FDA, Department of Health and Human Services [https://www.ecfr.gov/current/title-21]. In addition, the international ethical and scientific quality standard for designing, conducting, recording, and reporting trials that involve the participation of human subjects in accordance with Good Clinical Practice standards apply as outlined in the ICH E6 Good Clinical Practice guideline [https://www.ich.org/page/efficacy-guidelines].

3.2.2 US FDA Breakthrough Therapy Designation (BTD)

Breakthrough Therapy Designation was created by the US Congress under Section 902 of the 2012 Food and Drug Administration Safety and Innovation Act (FDASIA). This designation is rewarded to a drug that shows preliminary clinical evidence that the drug may demonstrate "substantial improvement over existing therapies on one or more clinically significant endpoints, such as substantial treatment effects observed early in clinical development." The clinical evidence to support a BTD is preliminary, and the FDA will review full data submitted to support approval and confirm that the drug ultimately is shown to demonstrate substantial improvement over existing therapies. If the designation is not supported by subsequent data, the FDA may rescind the designation to ensure that resources are focused on drugs that fulfill the BTD program qualifying criteria [https://www.fda.gov/regulatory-information/selected-amendments-fdc-act/food-and-drug-administration-safety-and-innovation-act-fdasia].

3.2.3 US FDA Regenerative Medicine Advanced Therapy (RMAT) Designation

The US Congress, under Section 3033 of the 21st Century Cures Act of 2016, authorized the FDA CBER to develop guidance for expedited programs for regenerative medicine therapies (RMAT) for serious conditions in recognition of the expanding field of regenerative medicine therapies. Guidance for the qualifying criteria for RMAT designation was published in 2019 to ensure such therapies are licensed and available to patients as soon as it can be established that these therapies are safe and effective. RMATs are eligible for other FDA-expedited programs, including FT and BTD, as well as PR and AA if they meet the criteria for any of these programs. As with other therapies that have expedited program designations, these therapies must meet the evidentiary standards for any approval, accelerated or traditional, by demonstrating effectiveness and safety.

Consistent with all FDA-expedited programs, information that supports more than one designation can be submitted in each separate designation request. In the case of RMAT designation, the FDA CBER expects preliminary clinical evidence will be part of the application and will demonstrate the potential of the regenerative medicine therapy to address the unmet medical need. There is flexibility to use clinical evidence obtained from clinical investigations using appropriately chosen historical controls or evidence from well-designed retrospective studies or clinical case series, as long as the preliminary clinical evidence is generated using the RMAT product that the sponsor intends to use for clinical development. Unlike the BTD, the RMAT designation does not require evidence to indicate the drug may offer substantial improvement over available therapies. Criteria for submission of the RMAT designation request can be found in the guidance [https:// www.fda.gov/vaccines-blood-biologics/cellular-gene-therapy-products/ regenerative-medicine-advanced-therapy-designation].

Definitions of a serious disease or condition, unmet medical need, surrogate endpoint, intermediate clinical endpoint (ICE), and clinically significant endpoint have the same meanings and interpretations in the guidance for all expedited programs. In its assessments for these designations, when preliminary clinical evidence is required, the FDA considers factors such as rigor of data collection, consistency and interpretability of outcomes, number of patients evaluated that contribute to the data, and the severity, rarity, or prevalence of the disease or condition. As with all reviews of small amounts of clinical data, the FDA pays particular attention to the potential for bias in study design, treatment assignment, or outcome assessment that could factor into the interpretation of the data. Careful attention to the control of such bias is an important consideration, and early consultation with the Office of Tissues and Advanced Therapies within the FDA CBER is encouraged to align the elements of early product development before such data are generated and submitted.

3.2.4 US FDA Priority Review (PR)

Prior to approval, each drug intended for registration in the United States must go through a thorough review by the responsible center division in the FDA. In 1992, under the Prescription Drug User Act, the FDA agreed to specific goals for improving the drug review cycle time and created two review timelines – *standard review* and *priority review (PR)*. The PR designation, with criteria for a completed review of an application within 6 months, satisfied the intent to direct resources to the evaluation of drugs that, if approved, would offer significant improvements in the safety, effectiveness of treatment, diagnosis, or prevention of serious conditions when compared with standard applications. An applicant may request PR, and the FDA informs the applicant of a designation within 60 days of the submission of the original BLA, NDA, or efficacy supplement. It is important to note that a PR designation does not alter the scientific standard for approval or the quality of evidence necessary for the regulatory decision.

3.2.5 US FDA Accelerated Approval (AA)

In 1992, the FDA instituted its AA program to allow for the earlier approval of drugs that treat serious conditions and that fill an unmet medical need based on a *surrogate endpoint or intermediate clinical endpoint*. It is important to consider that the default position for any product approval is to follow a standard development plan pursuing traditional approval and that a rationale for why traditional approval is not an option should be substantiated in plans to pursue an AA strategy (e.g., feasibility due to small sample size of the disease, or inability to collect clinical outcome measures in a reasonable period of time due to the natural history of the disease or condition). Expect regulators to push back on a proposal of accelerated/conditional approval, especially early in development if there is insufficient justification for not pursuing a standard development option. In general, the decision to accept a surrogate endpoint or ICE for AA is data-driven and considered case by case.

A *surrogate endpoint* is defined as a marker such as a laboratory measurement (biomarker), radiographic image, physical sign, or other measure that is likely to predict clinical benefit but is not itself a measure of clinical benefit. An *intermediate clinical endpoint* is a clinical endpoint that may be measured earlier than survival or irreversible morbidity. The acceptance of a *surrogate endpoint* or *ICE* can considerably shorten the time required prior to receiving marketing approval. Importantly, AA is a full approval, based on the scientific evidence in the application. There are limitations to product labeling in the United States at the time of approval, and the sponsor is still required to conduct studies to confirm the anticipated clinical benefit. Final evidence of clinical benefit is required to be submitted to the FDA as an efficacy supplement to support the conversion to traditional approval and additional product labeling. Should the confirmatory trials for clinical benefit fail to demonstrate that the drug is effective, the FDA has regulatory procedures in place that could lead to the removal of the drug from the market.

3.2.6 US FDA Fast Track (FT)

In 1997, the FDA created the FT designation, designed to facilitate the development and expedite the review of drugs to treat serious conditions and fill an unmet medical need. FT designation offers more frequent meetings and/or written communications with the FDA to discuss the development plan and the proposed design of clinical trials and use of biomarkers. This assures the sponsor that questions and issues about the development program can be resolved quickly, thus potentially expediting development of the drug.

It also offers the opportunity for a *rolling review,* which means that completed sections of the NDA or BLA can be submitted to the FDA for review before the entire application is available.

More information on AA, FT, and PR can be accessed online at [https://www.fda.gov/patients/fast-track-breakthrough-therapy-accelerated-approval-priority-review/priority-review].

3.2.7 US Rare Pediatric Disease Priority Review Vouchers

The US Congress under Section 529 of the 2012 FDA Safety and Innovation Act also sought to encourage development of new therapies for the prevention and treatment of certain rare pediatric diseases by incentivizing sponsors with the award of a voucher that can be used to obtain PR for any subsequent human drug application of the sponsor's choosing submitted to the FDA after the date of approval of the rare pediatric disease drug. This incentive program complements other applicable programs, including orphan drug designation under the Orphan Drug Act for rare disease therapies, and programs that encourage or require the evaluation of a drug used in pediatric populations under the Pediatric Research Equity Act (PREA) [https://www.fda.gov/regulatory-information/search-fda-guidance-documents/how-comply-pediatric-research-equity-act] and the Best Pharmaceuticals for Children Act (BPCA), which confer pediatric marketing exclusivity incentives.

3.2.8 FDA Guidance for Drug Development on Specific Topics in Rare Disease

The US FDA has a number of guidance and draft guidance documents, and other regulatory guidance intended to inform sponsors of their current thinking on specific topics in drug development for rare disease and conditions. The reader is recommended to consult these documents for applicable guidance on relevant topics as a supplement to direct engagement meetings with FDA-applicable divisions early and throughout drug development. These include the following topics, keeping in mind that the FDA frequently revises and adds new draft guidance to assist sponsors in their research plans for addressing the unmet needs of patients with rare disease and conditions. Guidance below reflects the current state of both general and disease-specific thinking of the FDA on a number of rare disease and orphan disease topics. The reader is encouraged to consult the FDA Guidance website [https://www.fda.gov/drugs/guidance-compliance-regulatory-information/guidances-drugs] for the most current guidance on these and newer topics:

- Human Gene Therapy for Neurodegenerative Diseases (2021)
- Interpreting Sameness of Gene Therapy Products Under the Orphan Drug Regulations (2021)

- Interpreting Sameness of Monoclonal Antibody Products Under the Orphan Drug Regulations (2014)
- Meetings with the Office of Orphan Products Development: Guidance for Industry, Researchers, Patient Groups and FDA Staff (2015)
- Clarification of Orphan Designation of Drugs and Biologics for Pediatric Subpopulations of Common Diseases (2017) Guidance for Industry
- Guidance for Industry and FDA Staff - Humanitarian Use Device (HUD) Designations (2019) and Humanitarian Device Exemption (HDE) Program (2019)
- Demonstrating Substantial Evidence of Effectiveness for Human Drug and Biological Products (2019)
- Expedited Programs for Serious Conditions—Drugs and Biologics (2014)
- Providing Regulatory Submissions in Electronic Format Orphan-Drug and Humanitarian Use Device Designation Requests and Related Submissions: Draft Guidance for Industry (2006)
- Fabry Disease: Developing Drugs for Treatment Guidance for Industry (2019)
- Expedited Programs for Regenerative Medicine Therapies for Serious Conditions (2019)
- Human Gene Therapy for Hemophilia (2020)
- Human Gene Therapy for Rare Diseases: Guidance for Industry (2020)
- Rare Pediatric Disease Priority Review Vouchers: Draft Guidance for Industry (2019)
- Rare Diseases: Natural History Studies for Drug Development: Draft Guidance for Industry (2019)
- Rare Diseases: Common Issues in Drug Development Guidance for Industry (2019)
- Rare Diseases: Early Drug Development and the Role of Pre-IND Meetings: Draft Guidance for Industry (2018)
- Duchenne Muscular Dystrophy and Related Dystrophinopathies: Developing Drugs for Treatment Guidance for Industry (2018)
- Slowly Progressive, Low Prevalence Rare Diseases with Substrate Deposition that Results from Single Enzyme Defects: Providing Evidence of Effectiveness for Replacement of Corrective Therapies: Guidance for Industry (2018)
- Pediatric Rare Disease: A Collaborative Approach for Drug Development Using Gaucher Disease as a Model: Draft Guidance for Industry (2017)

For a general comprehensive guidance that covers the challenges and considerations in planning any drug development program in rare diseases, the reader may consult the FDA Guidance for Industry, Rare Diseases: Common Issues in Drug Development (2019) online at [https://www.fda.gov/regulatory-information/search-fda-guidance-documents/rare-diseases-common-issues-drug-development-guidance-industry]. The recommendations and considerations outlined in this guidance will provide an understanding of expectations from the US FDA for elements of a rare disease drug development program to support evidence generation necessary for regulatory decision-making.

It is important to keep in mind that regulatory guidance and requirements, including nonclinical, clinical, and quality requirements, for the development of any single or complex drug, biologic, cellular, or gene therapy product, also apply to development of products for rare diseases and conditions.

3.3 EMA Guidance and Tools for Drug Development in Rare Disease

Similar to the FDA, the EMA provides regulatory guidance and incentives for research and development of medicines for rare diseases in the EU. Information on these policies and procedures is available on the EMA website under Human regulatory, Research and Development at EMA [https://www.ema.europa.eu/en/human-regulatory/research-development/orphan-designation-research-development].

Although the EMA does not publish specific guidance documents for rare disease drug development, there is guidance available on the EMA website pertaining to the relevant topics, including advanced therapy classification, orphan designation, accelerated assessment, conditional marketing authorization, pediatric medicines, PRIME, scientific advice and protocol assistance, procedural advice and guidance on CHMP/CAT/PRAC, guidance on technical document and data standards, and support for early access.

Similar to the FDA, the EMA adheres to harmonized regulatory guidance in the efficacy, safety, quality, and multidisciplinary guidelines adopted by the ICH.

3.3.1 EMA Orphan Designation

In line with the requirements of Article 3, the EU Orphan Regulation (EC) No 141/2000, the Committee for Orphan Medicinal Products (COMP) evaluates applications for orphan designation according to the following criteria:

- The medicine must be intended for the treatment, prevention, or diagnosis of a disease that is life-threatening or chronically debilitating.

- The prevalence of the condition in the EU must not be more than 5 in 10,000, or it must be unlikely that marketing the medicine would generate sufficient returns to justify the investment of development cost.
- There are no approved satisfactory therapies available for the diagnosis, prevention, or treatment of the condition, or the intended new medicine offers significant benefit over existing therapies.

It is important to note that the EMA and the FDA have different prevalence thresholds on what is considered "rare" or "orphan". In addition, in the EU, the sponsor must demonstrate that the medicine confers a significant benefit in the condition compared with existing therapies. The assessment of a significant benefit over existing therapies can be demonstrated in several ways, including improved efficacy and/or safety, or in the case where a drug works as well as existing treatments, it should represent a major contribution to patient care.

Orphan designation in the EU offers a 10-year market exclusivity period upon marketing authorization as an incentive for drug development support. Applications for Orphan designation can be submitted to the EMA at any time during drug development before the marketing authorization application (MAA) is submitted. Early designation in development offers additional guidance and support by the EMA, including protocol assistance, a type of scientific advice specific for designated orphan medicines.

For further access to EU law, the reader is referred to https://eur-lex.europa.eu/homepage.html.

3.3.2 EMA PRIority MEdicines (PRIME) Scheme

PRIME was launched by the EMA in 2016 to enhance support for drug development of medicines that target an unmet medical need [https://www.ema.europa.eu/en/human-regulatory/research-development/prime-priority-medicines]. Similar to the FDA BTD and RMAT, eligibility for PRIME requires preliminary clinical evidence of the promise of a new medicine, except for the academic sector and small enterprises that can access the scheme on the basis of compelling nonclinical data and tolerability data from initial clinical trials. This is a voluntary program with the benefit of early and enhanced dialogue with the EMA to optimize development and accelerate evaluation. Early appointment of a rapporteur from the Committee for Medicinal Products for Human Use (CHMP) or the Committee for Advanced Therapies (CAT), a kick-off meeting with the CHMP/CAT rapporteur and a multidisciplinary group of experts, scientific advice at key development milestones, and earlier involvement of health technology assessment bodies are all benefits of PRIME designation intended to help guide the overall development plan and regulatory strategy and facilitate quicker market access for patients upon marketing authorization.

PRIME builds on the existing regulatory framework at the EMA such as scientific advice and, at the time of marketing application, Accelerated Assessment.

3.3.3 EMA Advanced Therapies

The EMA can provide early guidance and support, including reduced fees, for advanced therapy medicinal products (ATMPs) for human use that are based on genes, tissues, or cells acknowledging that these offer "groundbreaking new opportunities for the treatment of disease or injury" [https://www.ema.europa.eu/en/human-regulatory/overview/advanced-therapy-medicinal-products-overview]. ATMPs are classified into three main categories: gene therapy medicines, somatic cell therapy medicines, and tissue-engineered medicines. In addition, this classification includes combined ATMPs, for example, cells encased in a bioengineered scaffold. These programs are under the guidance of the EMA CAT. The CAT plays a crucial role in the scientific assessment of an ATMP and provides its opinion on the quality, safety, and efficacy of the product to the CHMP for consideration by the CHMP in its recommendation or not for the authorization of the medicine.

3.3.4 EU Centralized Procedure and Accelerated Assessment

The EU pharmaceutical legislation includes provisions for granting expedited review to new medicines of major interest to public health such as serious and life-threatening conditions, including rare diseases. Under the centralized procedure, sponsors can submit their MAA to the EMA as a single EU submission for scientific assessment. If authorization is granted, the centralized marketing authorization is valid in all EU member states and the European Economic Area (EEA) countries of Iceland, Liechtenstein, and Norway. It is important to remember that since the United Kingdom withdrawal from the EU in 2020, the United Kingdom is no longer covered by the EMA process. Engagements on the acceptability of drug development programs in support of an intended marketing authorization submission in the United Kingdom, therefore, must be directed to the Medicines and Healthcare products Regulatory Agency (MHRA). Given the independence of the MHRA, it is recommended to have discussions with the MHRA early to ensure all elements to support a marketing authorization in the United Kingdom are considered in the development program.

Accelerated assessment reduces the timeframe for the EMA to review an MAA. The standard timeframe for a review of an MAA submitted under the centralized procedure can take up to 210 days, not counting when applicants may need to provide additional information at the CHMP request. If the application is deemed eligible for an accelerated assessment, the time for CHMP review and action can be reduced to 150 days. An application for consideration of *accelerated assessment* typically takes place 2–3 months before the planned MAA.

3.3.5 EU Conditional Marketing Authorization

In the interests of public health, especially in seriously debilitating or life-threatening disease, including rare/orphan diseases or conditions where no alternative therapies exist and where the benefit of immediate availability of the medicine outweighs the risk, an application may be granted a *conditional marketing authorization (MA)* based on less comprehensive clinical data than normally required for a full approval. Conditional marketing authorizations are valid for 1 year and can be renewed annually. The MA holder is required to fulfil specific obligations within defined timelines, which typically include completing ongoing or new studies or collecting additional data to confirm that the benefit-risk profile of the drug remains positive. Once confirmed that the required specific obligations and data are comprehensive, the conditional MA can be converted into a standard marketing authorization.

3.4 Other Global Regulatory Considerations in Drug Development for Rare and Orphan Diseases

3.4.1 Compassionate Use

Both the FDA and EMA have provisions for the compassionate use of unapproved/unauthorized medicines. Under specific agreements and conditions, compassionate use programs are reserved for those patients with seriously debilitating disease or life-threatening diseases that are not satisfactorily treated and who are unable or ineligible to participate in ongoing clinical trials.

In the United States, the FDA has issued guidance on Expanded Access to Investigational Drugs for Treatment Use for individual patients or patient populations through a treatment IND or treatment protocol [https://www.fda.gov/news-events/public-health-focus/expanded-access]. US regulations describe criteria that must be met to authorize expanded access use that include safeguards intended to protect the rights and safety of patients and preserve the ability to develop meaningful data about the safety and effectiveness of the drug as evaluations continue under the IND through clinical trials. Expanded access INDs and protocols are generally not designed to determine the efficacy of a drug as they typically involve uncontrolled exposures with limited data collection; however, the expanded access regulations in the United States do not prohibit the collection of such data.

In the EU, compassionate use programs are generally coordinated and implemented through member states, which set their own rules and procedures. The medicine must be undergoing clinical trials or have entered the marketing authorization procedure.

3.4.2 Pediatric Rare Disease

If the rare disease or condition includes or is limited to pediatric patients, then plans for evaluation of the drug in the relevant pediatric population are required by both the FDA and EMA.

For all drug development, regardless of indication, both the FDA and EMA have specific laws and regulations governing the development of drugs for the pediatric population, unless criteria are met for a drug-specific or class waiver. Importantly, the requirement for pediatric studies differs by region; therefore, the legislation and procedures relevant for pediatric drug development, including timelines for submission of clinical study plans, requests for waivers and/or deferrals, and timing for completion of studies and submission of results for review, are specific to US and EU agencies. These requirements are not limited to orphan or rare diseases but apply to all drug development programs for pediatric populations.

Both the FDA and EMA abide by the principles outlined in ICH E11 and its updates: Clinical Investigation of Medicinal Products in the Pediatric Population, and principles for Pediatric Extrapolation of data to support pediatric drug development [https://www.ich.org/page/efficacy-guidelines].

3.4.2.1 US Pediatric Drug Development

In the United States, there are two cornerstone pediatric drug development laws:

- Pediatric Research Equity Act (PREA)
- Best Pharmaceuticals for Children Act (BPCA)

PREA [https://www.fda.gov/drugs/development-resources/pediatric-research-equity-act-prea] requires companies to assess safety and effectiveness of new drugs/biologics/therapies in pediatric patients. PREA requires mandatory studies only on the indication(s) under review if they apply to pediatric patients and adults. If the indication pertains exclusively to adults or if other criteria are met, studies in the pediatric population may be granted a full (all pediatric ages) or partial (a subset of pediatric population) *waiver*. Under PREA, current laws exempt the mandatory studies for orphan-designated indications, but this could be subject to future change, as in the development of drugs for orphan adult oncology indications where the PREA waiver have been rescinded by law (the Research to Accelerate Cures and Equity for Children Act enacted 2017) to expand treatment options for pediatric cancer patients by mandating that all new adult oncology drugs also be tested in children when the molecular targets are relevant to a particular childhood cancer.

All data in PREA studies are intended to inform labeling for the pediatric population. PREA requirements are triggered by an application for a new indication, new dosage form or dosing regimen, new route of administration, or a new active ingredient for an adult population. For drugs that fall under the PREA requirement, a pediatric study plan is required within 60 days of the end of phase 2 meeting with the FDA, or no later than 210 days prior to the intended submission of the application. With FDA agreement, the submission of some or all assessments of pediatric drug safety and efficacy may be *deferred* until a specified time after approval of the drug for adult use (e.g., until additional safety or efficacy data have been collected in adults). As noted above, with justification, certain pediatric subgroups (e.g., neonates) may be *waived*.

The BPCA [https://www.fda.gov/drugs/development-resources/best-pharmaceuticals-children-act-bpca] provides a financial incentive to companies to *voluntarily* conduct pediatric studies under a written request (WR) from the FDA. A sponsor may request the FDA to issue a WR by submitting a proposed pediatric study request. Studies may be requested for orphan indications where there is no PREA requirement for development in children. Under the BPCA, studies required to satisfy the granting of the incentive of additional months of marketing exclusivity relate to the entire moiety and may expand indications beyond that being studied in the adult population (approved and/or unapproved indications). In addition, under the BPCA, neonates must be addressed in the WR. Exclusivity attaches to all existing marketing exclusivities and patents for the drug moiety and does not require positive pediatric studies (although the clinical data must be interpretable). Granting of exclusivity is reviewed by the FDA Pediatric Exclusivity Board.

The ultimate goal of PREA and the BPCA is new pediatric labeling to encourage and ensure the appropriate use of medicines to treat pediatric patients.

3.4.2.2 EU Pediatric Drug Development

The EU Pediatric Regulation, (EC) No 1901/2006, was authorized in January 2007 [https://www.ema.europa.eu/en/human-regulatory/overview/paediatric-medicines/paediatric-regulation] with the objective to improve the health of children in the EU. This regulation ensures that medicines developed for use in children are of high quality, ethically researched, and authorized appropriately with the goal of improving both access and information on their appropriate use.

MAA for new drugs not authorized in the EU must include the results of studies conducted in the pediatric population, in compliance with an agreed pediatric investigation plan (PIP), unless the EMA has granted a deferral or waiver. Deferrals are granted if there are insufficient data to demonstrate the efficacy and safety of the drug in adults. Waivers are granted when pediatric development is not needed or not appropriate. Once authorization is obtained, study results are included in labeling (even if negative), and the drug is eligible for additional supplementary protection certificate extension. For orphan-designated products, the 10-year period of market exclusivity is extended to

12 years. These extensions also apply to authorized medicines when a new indication (including pediatric) is added, or a new formulation or new route of administration is approved. If the medication is exclusive to the pediatric population with age appropriate formulations, a pediatric-use marketing authorization is incentivized with a 10-year period of data/market protection.

The PIP must be agreed in advance by the EMA Paediatric Committee (PDCO), including elements of protocol design and formulation to generate data to support the pediatric indication in all relevant pediatric age-groups. The PDCO will engage with other EMA committees on any matters related to the development program for pediatric use.

To advance the global development of medicines for children, both EMA and the US FDA have agreed on principles for interaction and exchange of information on pediatric matters. Regulators responsible for guiding pediatric drug development within the FDA Pediatric Review Committee and EMA PDCO have regular discussions in the context of cluster activities in an effort to coordinate a common approach to pediatric drug development considering that regional legislation adheres to different timelines for meeting pediatric requirements. This ensures that during drug development for pediatric populations, a sponsor has the opportunity to meet both regional requirements in the EMA Pediatric Investigation Plan (PIP) and in the US Pediatric Study Plan. All expedited approaches in both agencies are available for rare disease pediatric drug development.

3.5 Overall Considerations in Rare Disease Drug Development

In summary, although the statutory requirements for the demonstration of efficacy and safety are not unique to rare disease drug development, regulatory agencies can exercise flexibility in their scientific judgement in determining the level of evidence a sponsor is required to provide to support a marketing application for a drug intended to treat a rare disease. It is acknowledged by regulators that these development programs are more challenging due to limitations in medical and scientific knowledge and natural history data, and/or regulatory precedent for established and validated surrogate biomarkers, clinical outcome assessments, and endpoints and by the limitations of conducting clinical studies in small populations of patients with high unmet medical needs, often with a willingness to accept a balance of risks versus benefit when there are inferior or absent treatment options. It is universally encouraged by global regulatory authorities that sponsors seek early and continued engagement with regulators to ensure that their development programs will meet the requirements for expedited and early access regulatory pathways and programs and have the greatest potential to bring new therapies to patients.

4

Clinical Trial Design and Analysis Considerations for Rare Diseases

Lanju Zhang, Lingyun Liu, Bingming Yi, Xiaopeng Miao, Nitin Nair, Xiaoyan Liu, Ina Jazic, and Glen Laird

Vertex Pharmaceuticals

Xiaolong Luo

Sarepta Pharmaceuticals

CONTENTS

DOI: 10.1201/9781003080954-4

4.1 General Considerations

Rare diseases are those with a relatively low frequency of affected patients in the general population. For example, a disease is considered rare if less than 1 out of 2,000 in the EU, 1,500 in the US and 2,500 in Japan is affected. Rare diseases have been under-researched; therefore, usually, there is a high unmet medical need. Recent advance in biology, genetics and genomic sciences, and technology has enabled a wave of possibilities for treating such diseases. For example, gene editing is particularly efficient in treating rare diseases caused by a single gene mutation.

Approval of rare disease treatments requires a favorable benefit–risk profile similar to prevalent disease treatments. However, due to the limited patient population, the justification of a favorable benefit–risk profile may be different. For example, instead of following through the typical phase I, phase II, and phase III development paradigm, a rare disease treatment development program may only include a single trial, sometimes even with a single arm. In addition, a rare disease treatment registration typically does not require two confirmatory, controlled, and randomized trials to provide adequate evidence.

However, the primary principles of clinical trial designs are still needed. Some diseases still require randomized and controlled trials for registration. In this case, group sequential designs, sometimes with sample size re-estimation, are applicable. In other situations, to deal with the challenge of the limited patient population, atypical designs, such as a crossover design, enrichment design, or N of 1 design should be considered. From the whole development program perspective, seamless designs and master protocol designs can bring significant efficiency.

In this chapter, we will start with some considerations on endpoint selection. Then, we will move on to introduce different trial designs and analysis methods, with an emphasis on applications in rare disease treatment development. Rare disease trial examples are provided for many designs.

4.2 Some Considerations on Endpoint Selection in Rare Disease Trials

In the design of clinical trials, it is critical to identify and select endpoints that can effectively differentiate the outcomes between patients with the intervention and those without, and these outcomes should be clinically meaningful for patients' benefits. For clinical trials in prevalent diseases, substantial prior research and pharmaceutical development have often been conducted, leading to regulatory precedents for endpoint selection. By the nature of rare diseases, there is often limited medical and scientific knowledge, natural history data, and drug development experiences. Many developers are literally pioneers in the area and there are often no well-characterized efficacy endpoints available. However, the need still exists to identify and select endpoints that are assessable and can likely demonstrate the experimental drug's effectiveness, if any, for regulatory approval.

Given the overwhelming unmet need in patients with rare diseases, there is always the desire and urgency to deliver a successful trial early and bring the benefit of medical innovation to patients. Endpoint selection has a large impact on the logistics of clinical trial conduct and success. While it is relatively easy to collect short-term endpoints, they may or may not translate to patients' ultimate long-term clinical benefit. In addition, some treatments may take time to be differentially effective. While long-term or longitudinal endpoints allow a complete assessment of patients' health trajectory, it can be logistically challenging and impactful on trial quality with heterogeneous and sometimes missing data. In addition, for randomized studies on rare diseases, it is not always ethical for patients to stay in an untreated group for an extended period while switching treatment early may reduce the power of the trial.

Fortunately, we are in a digital era with technology making electronic health records and real-world data readily available. There are often observational studies for many diseases. There are many *consortia* and initiatives that focus on individual diseases. For example, the COMET Initiative (https://www.comet-initiative.org/) provides a rich resource of searchable databases. TREAT-NMD, a network for the neuromuscular field, aims to collate information about existing outcome measures into a single and freely available online resource. Some lead investigators have the expertise and maintain studies of the natural history of diseases in the area. Advisory committees formed by those experts provide relevant and practical opinions on initial endpoints that are relevant to patients with a preliminary characterization of their variation that are critical for sample size assessment. Given the high heterogeneity of many rare diseases and the observational approach of natural history studies or registries, it is important to properly integrate and analyze anecdotal findings and incorporate them into a trial design that accounts for a likely unknown confounding effect.

A common limitation in conducting rare disease trials is the lack of sufficient patients for enrollment. There is thus more consideration in optimizing the choice of the endpoint to improve trial enrollment. Two areas that warrant special attention are intra-subject experimental units and transitional endpoints.

In the context of the design of clinical trials, we usually consider one subject as an experimental unit. When a subject is assessed longitudinally, there are multiple measurements per subject. Under some conditions, these measurements may be approximately independent and can be seen as intra-subject experimental units that capture the treatment effect. In a study published by Harmatz et al. (2018) that investigated vestronidase alfa for mucopolysaccharidosis VII, an ultra-rare genetic disease, subjects were randomized 1:1:1:1 to one of four treatment sequence groups to either 4 mg/kg vestronidase alfa (Group A) or placebo and crossover to 4 mg/kg vestronidase alfa at predefined time points (Weeks 8, 16, and 24 for Groups B, C, and D, respectively). Subjects were assessed for urinary GAG (uGAG) excretion from baseline to Week 24. The data was analyzed by a general estimating equation (GEE) model, including baseline value as a covariate and the week after active treatment as a fixed effect. It can be noted, that if the assumption that weekly assessments are independent for each subject is appropriate, the GEE model technically implements all weekly assessments as experimental units, mitigating the limited sample size. We cite this example only for illustrative purposes. In real cases, biological and clinical input should be taken into consideration for the relevant statistical model assumption.

In a more general approach, we can view the longitudinal assessments of one or more endpoints as transitional states and evaluate relevant outcomes through its transition function (Baghfalaki and Ganjali, 2020). With appropriate modeling of these transitional states and covariates, we can aggregate intra-subject sequential data to evaluate the relationship between treatments and outcomes from early and late stages. This view includes the more commonly described concept of surrogate endpoint but is more general. Even with one endpoint, there is often interest in evaluating the outcome at different time points and the predictability of the later outcome based on the earlier outcome. Thus, early assessment can be viewed as a potential "surrogate endpoint."

There has been a rich body of research on surrogate endpoints. A frequently quoted definition of a surrogate endpoint is from Section 506(c) of the Federal Food, Drug, and Cosmetic Act 272 (FD&C Act) that FDA may grant accelerated approval to

> a product for a serious or life-threatening disease or condition ... upon a determination that the product has an effect on a surrogate endpoint that is reasonably likely to predict clinical benefit, or on a clinical endpoint that can be measured earlier than irreversible morbidity or mortality, that is reasonably likely to predict an effect on irreversible morbidity or mortality or other clinical benefit.

In the context of innovation theorem (Andersen et al., 1991) and based on the assumption of invariant innovated transition function of the clinical endpoint from surrogate endpoints, Prentice (1989) provides a technically sufficient condition to quantify the clause of "reasonably likely to predict clinical benefit". While the assumption simplifies the concept of a surrogate endpoint, it may not be held in practice or necessary either. With the modern technology of data science, we can utilize neuron network construct to approximate the transition function directly and characterize the predictability of early endpoint profile on the primary endpoint in later clinical benefit. Such deep learning can be learned from early trial results as well as natural history and real-world evidence data. In the area of rare diseases, many experimental drugs are proposed with biological rationale and supported by early research. It is compelling to learn and utilize the outcome transition function from those biological findings and optimize the cost of trial conduct as well as the efficiency to effectively differentiate the experimental drug effect. A recent example is Tardivon et al (2019).

4.3 Design and Analysis of Clinical Trials for Rare Diseases

In this section, we introduce typical trial designs used for rare disease treatment development.

4.3.1 Group Sequential and Sample Size Reestimation Designs for Rare Disease Trials

4.3.1.1 Introduction

In the traditional clinical trial design, the sample size is often determined to detect the target treatment effect with adequate power. However, it is not always easy to define the target treatment effect size. The treatment effect is typically estimated based on limited prior trial data and thus admits to large uncertainties while a clinically meaningful difference may be difficult to determine in a rare disease. If the effect size is overestimated, the sample size could be too small resulting in an underpowered study. On the other hand, the sample size could be too large leading to an overpowered study if the effect size is underestimated at the design stage. Trial designs are even more complex for rare diseases due to (1) a small patient population, (2) a heterogeneous patient population (e.g., different genotypes), and (3) poor characterization of the disease.

EMA (2006) and FDA (2019a) have published guidances (EMA Guideline on Clinical Trials in Small Populations; FDA Guidance for Rare Diseases: Common Issues in Drug Development Guidance for Industry) to discuss these issues and what sponsors should consider addressing these issues in drug development for rare diseases. In both guidances, adaptive designs are referenced as one of the approaches to gain efficiency for drug development in rare diseases. There are many types of adaptive designs developed in the literature to handle different risks or uncertainties about the trials in the confirmatory setting; among which, group sequential designs and sample size reestimation designs are the most adopted ones in the pharmaceutical industry to address the uncertainty related to the treatment effect (or standardized effect). The philosophy behind group sequential designs is to target a small and conservative treatment effect with large sample size, with one or more interim analyses built in to cut down the sample size if overwhelming efficacy is observed in the interim. Statistically valid methods have been established to design and analyze group sequential designs to ensure strong control of type I error rate and appropriate power under the range of treatment effect size of interest. The range of treatment effects of interest is often between the minimum clinically meaningful treatment effect, which is often determined by the available standard of care (SOC), the therapeutic landscape and other factors for market access, and the best effect sponsors could hope for based on existing data on the drug candidates. The fundamental theory for group sequential designs is developed by Scharfstein et al. (1997) and Jennison and Turnbull (2000) where they showed the joint distribution of the Wald statistics computed sequentially at each interim look is asymptotically multivariate normal with a canonical distribution. Such canonical distributions are the backbone for deriving the efficacy/futility stopping boundaries to ensure the type I error rate control and target power. The commonly used boundaries to monitor trials with group sequential designs are based on spending functions such as Lan and DeMets (1983). For rare disease patient populations, asymptotic distributions often do not hold, especially with binary outcomes. In the next section, we will use an example in severe sickle cell disease to illustrate how to design trials in rare diseases with binary outcomes.

Group sequential design is an efficient method to address the uncertainty of the treatment effect at the design stage. However, group sequential design is not always feasible since it might be challenging for the sponsor to decide how small a treatment effect should be targeted at the design stage. The smallest clinically meaningful treatment effect is often not well defined for rare diseases since there is typically little to no data in the literature. A more flexible design to mitigate the risk of uncertainty about treatment effect at the design stage is to allow sample size adaptation in addition to early stopping for efficacy or futility. Trials could start with a smaller sample size targeting a more optimistic treatment effect. In the interim, data can be reviewed to check if a sample size increase is warranted to increase the likelihood of success. This type of design is especially appealing for rare disease trials whose sponsors are often biotechnology companies with trial budgets dependent on trial milestones. A few approaches have been proposed to control the type I error rate in case of sample size adaptation based on an unblinded sample size reestimation. These methods include Cui et al. (1999), Lehmacher and Wassmer (1999), Chen et al. (2004); Müller and Schäfer (2001); Mehta and Pocock (2011). A clinical trial in patients with Takayasu arteritis (TAK) will be used as an example to illustrate the idea and benefit of adaptive sample size reestimation.

4.3.1.2 Exact Group Sequential Design for a Clinical Trial in Sickle Cell Disease

Sickle cell disease is a rare genetic blood disorder that affects the structure and function of hemoglobin, reduces the ability of red blood cells to transport oxygen efficiently, and progresses to a chronic vascular disease. Consider a single-arm clinical trial in a subpopulation of severe sickle cell disease. The primary endpoint is severe vaso-occlusive crisis (VOC) free for at least 12 consecutive months. For this severe subpopulation, the 12-month VOC-free response rate for SOC is assumed to be 60%. The new therapy is expected to increase the rate to 80%. It is desired to design a three-look group sequential design with 90% power at a one-sided 0.025 level. The intention of the interim looks is to align with early submission for the approval of new treatment. Let p denote the proportion of subjects with VOC free for at least 12 consecutive months, $p_0 = 0.6$ denote the rate for SOC, and $p_1 = 0.8$ denote the rate for the new treatment. Hypothesis testing can be formulated as the null hypothesis $H_0 : p = p_0$ and one-sided alternative $H_1 : p > p_0$. We are targeting the specific alternative $p = p_1$. Let's first consider a group sequential design based on the asymptotic test. Let Z_k $(k = 1,2,3)$ denote the cumulative Wald statistics at each look defined as follows:

$$Z_k = \frac{\hat{p}_k - p_0}{\sqrt{\dfrac{p_0(1-p_0)}{n_k}}}$$

where $\hat{p}_k$ is the estimate of p based on the accumulative number of patients, n_k, at the look k. The asymptotic test would reject the null hypothesis if $Z_k > c_k$ where the asymptotic boundary c_k is typically constructed using error-spending functions. The boundary is calculated to satisfy the following equations at each look:

$$P(Z_1 > c_1) = \alpha_1$$

$$P(Z_1 \leq c_1, Z_2 > c_2) = \alpha_2 - \alpha_1$$

$$P(Z_1 \leq c_1, Z_2 \leq c_2, Z_3 > c_3) = \alpha - \alpha_1 - \alpha_2$$

where α_1, α_2 are the cumulative type I error rate spent at Look 1 and Look 2, α is the total type I error rate. For example, the stopping boundary with equal spacing based on O'Brien–Fleming spending function of Lan and DeMets (1983) is shown in Table 4.1 as 3.805, 2.478, and 1.996. The cumulative type I error rate spent at each look is shown as 0.00007, 0.007, and 0.025. Table 4.2 shows the boundary-crossing probabilities under H_0 and H_1 based on the asymptotic distribution versus the actual ones based on 100,000 simulations. Note that the simulated cumulative boundary-crossing probability under the null hypothesis is 0.04124 which is much larger than the nominal type I error rate of 0.025. Also, the simulated probability under H_1 is only 0.798 which is lower than the target power of 90%. The inflation of the type I error rate and loss of power are due to the small sample size and the discreteness of the endpoint. To design the study with an appropriate type I error rate and target power, we need to use exact methods to account for the discreteness and small sample size.

The calculations for exact group sequential design were discussed in Jennison and Turnbull (2000). It was originally described in Schultz et al. (1973). In this section, the sickle cell disease example will be used to illustrate the design based on the exact test. Let n_1, n_2 and $n_3 = n$ be the cumulative sample size at each look where n is the total sample size. Let $R_1, R_2,$

TABLE 4.1

Efficacy Boundary and Boundary-Crossing Probabilities based on Asymptotic Tests

Look #	Sample Size	Cumulative	Efficacy Boundary (c_1, c_2, c_3)
1	7	0.00007	3.805
2	15	0.007	2.478
3	22	0.025	1.996

TABLE 4.2

Boundary-Crossing Probabilities based on Asymptotic Tests against Simulated Boundary-Crossing Probabilities

| | Asymptotic Tests | | Simulation | |
B>Look #	Under H_0	Under H_1	Under H_0	Under H_1
1	0.00007	0.025	0	0
2	0.007	0.593	0.02761	0.604
3	0.025	0.904	0.04124	0.798

and R_3 be the cumulative number of VOC free subjects by each look. The boundaries can be calculated to satisfy the boundary-crossing probabilities at each look iteratively.

At look 1, c_1 is computed by the equation below:

$$P_0(R_1 \geq c_1) \leq \alpha_1$$

where $P_0(.)$ denotes the probability evaluated under H_0.

After c_1 is determined, the boundary c_2 at the second look is computed by the following equation:

$$P_0(R_1 \geq c_1) + P_0(R_1 < c_1, R_2 \geq c_2) \leq \alpha_2$$

where R_i follows binomial distribution (n_i, p_0). Note that the second term in the above equation can be expressed as:

$$P_0(R_1 < c_1, R_2 \geq c_2) = \sum_{i=1}^{c_1} P_0(R_1 = i-1) P_0\left(R_{(2)} > c_2 - i\right)$$

where $R_{(2)}$ is the incremental number of VOC free subjects observed from the $n_2 - n_1$ subjects enrolled between Look 1 and Look 2 and $R_{(2)}$ follows a binomial distribution $(n_2 - n_1, p_0)$.

The boundary at the last look 3 can be computed similarly using the following equation after the boundaries for the previous looks are already determined:

$$P_0(R_1 \geq c_1) + P_0(R_1 < c_1, R_2 \geq c_2) + P_0(R_1 < c_1, R_2 < c_2, R_3 \geq c_3) \leq \alpha_3$$

The third term in the above equation can be computed as:

$$P_0(R_1 < c_1, R_2 < c_2, R_3 \geq c_3) = \sum_{i=1}^{c_1}\sum_{j=1}^{c_2} P_0(R_1 = i-1) P_0\left(R_{(2)} = j-i\right) P_0\left(R_{(3)} > c_3 - j\right)$$

where $R_{(3)}$ is the incremental number of subjects with VOC free from the $n_3 - n_2$ subjects enrolled between Look 2 and the last look.

Table 4.3 shows the cumulative type I error rate, efficacy boundary, and the boundary-crossing probabilities under H_0 and H_1 using O'Brien–Fleming-spending function for a three-look group sequential design with equal spacing.

Note that the boundary at Look 1 is not available. This is again due to the discreteness of the distribution. At Look 1, the most stringent boundary is to assume that all 12 subjects are responders. In this case, the type I error rate $P_0(R_1 \geq 12) = 0.00218$ which is still greater than the nominal alpha defined

TABLE 4.3

Efficacy Boundary and Boundary-Crossing Probabilities Based on
Exact Method with LD(OF) Spending Function Boundary

Look #	Sample Size	LD (OF) Spending Function Boundary	Efficacy Boundary	Boundary-Crossing Probabilities	
				H_0	H_1
1	12	0.0001035	NA	0	0
2	24	0.006	21	0.004	0.505
3	36	0.025	28	0.021	0.921

by the Lan-DeMets O'Brien–Fleming [LD(OF)]-spending function. Therefore, one should use the spending function to guide the boundary determination together with the exploration of interim timing based on the trial-and-error approach (Table 4.4).

Using the boundary based on Lan-DeMets Pocock [LD(PK)]-spending function, the final attained type I error rate is 0.021 and the power is 0.914 which are all computed based on the exact distribution described earlier in this section.

One unique feature of group sequential design based on the exact method is that there might be multiple designs that meet the type I error rate requirement and the power is close to the target. This is reflected in the power plot of the seesaw shape. Figure 4.1 shows the power plot versus sample size for an exact three-look group sequential design using LD(PK) boundary (the plot is generated using EAST® 6).

Table 4.5 shows three designs, all of which have type I error rates below the nominal level of 0.025 and power close to the target of 90%. When the sample size is increased from 33 (Design 1) to 36 (Design 2), the power drops from 89.5% to 86.5%. This is because the type I error rate is not exhausted due to the discreteness. The attained type I error rate is only 0.018 for Design 2. For sample size 37, the power is 91.4% with a higher attained type I error rate too.

TABLE 4.4

Efficacy Boundary and Boundary-Crossing Probabilities based on
Exact Method with LD(PK) Spending Function Boundary

Look #	Sample Size	LD (PK) Spending Function Boundary	Efficacy Boundary	Boundary-Crossing Probabilities	
				H_0	H_1
1	12	0.011	12/12	0.002	0.142
2	25	0.019	21/25	0.011	0.687
3	37	0.025	29/37	0.021	0.914

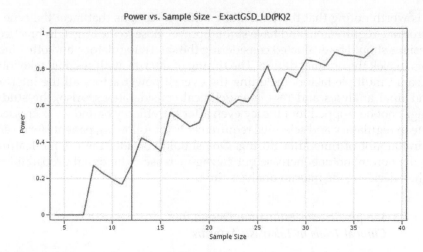

FIGURE 4.1
Power versus sample size for exact group sequential design based on Pocock error spending function of Lan and DeMets (1983).

TABLE 4.5

Three-Look Design with One-Sided Type I Error Rate 0.025 and Target Power 90%

	Design 1	Design 2	Design 3
Sample Size	33	36	37
Look timing and boundary at Look 1, 2, 3	11/11	12/12	12/12
	19/22	20/24	21/25
	26/33	29/36	29/37
Type I error rate	0.0239	0.018	0.0207
Power	0.895	0.865	0.914

Group sequential designs are more flexible designs compared to traditional fixed sample designs. They are more ethical by allowing early stopping for efficacy and futility for an overwhelming treatment effect or early signal of null effect. Although we didn't consider futility stopping for this trial, the futility boundary can be constructed similarly using the spending function approach or based on conditional power. The asymptotic theory for group sequential design breaks down for rare populations where the sample size is typically very small. As a result, the type I error rate might be inflated, or power might be compromised. Exact methods are needed to account for the exact distributions of the trial data. For trials with a binary outcome, group sequential tests can be constructed directly based on the number of responders at each look. Such a sequence of the number of responders has correlated binomial distributions. The efficacy boundary can be obtained using the exact binomial distributions to preserve the type I error rate.

It is worth noting that there might be multiple designs that meet the type I error rate requirement and have similar power close to the target. In practice, designs should be evaluated considering the safety, regulatory, and other factors to pick the optimal design. The timing of interim analyses may take into account multiple factors including the overall power across all the interim and final analyses and regulatory/clinical considerations. Also, the study might not be stopped for efficacy even after the efficacy boundary is crossed due to regulatory and scientific requirements for following patients for a certain amount of time after dosing. One should consider the unique feature of the non-monotone increase but zigzag increase of binomial probabilities, when deciding the interim analysis time.

4.3.1.3 Sample Size Re-Estimation Design for Clinical Trials in Takayasu Arteritis

TAK is a rare type of vasculitis that causes blood vessel inflammation. Such inflammation damages the large artery which carries blood from the heart to the rest of the body. It can also affect the major artery branches, coronary arteries, and pulmonary arteries. The estimated incidence is 2.6 per million in the United States and 60 per million in Japan. The tocilizumab in Takayasu arteritis (TAKT) study is a double-blind, placebo-controlled, multicenter trial designed to evaluate the steroid-sparing effect of tocilizumab. The primary endpoint was time to relapse of TAK according to protocol-defined criteria. The study planned to enroll 34 patients and accrue 19 events of relapse which would yield 90% of the power to detect a hazard ratio of 0.2075 at a two-sided alpha level of 0.05 assuming a relapse-free rate of 75% in the tocilizumab group and 25% in the placebo group at Week 24. An interim analysis for efficacy and futility was performed after 13 events of relapse. O'Brien–Fleming alpha- and beta-spending functions were used to monitor the trial in the interim and final analyses to preserve the overall type I error rate and power. Interim results were reviewed by the independent data monitoring committee (DMC). Neither the efficacy nor futility criteria were met in the interim. The trial continued to the end and a final analysis was conducted when 19 events of relapse were observed. The two-sided nominal p-value boundary at the final analysis was 0.0459.

The primary endpoint, time-to-relapse of TAK, was estimated using Kaplan–Meier analysis and log-rank test stratified by age category. The hazard ratio and corresponding confidence interval for tocilizumab compared to placebo were estimated using the Cox regression model stratified by age category. At the final analysis, the estimated relapse-free rates at week 24 were 50.6% for tocilizumab and 22.9% for placebo. The estimated hazard ratio for the time-to-relapse of TAK was 0.41 with a confidence interval (0.15, 1.10) and the p-value is 0.0596. The primary endpoint was not met since there was no significant difference between tocilizumab and placebo. However, the results on the per-protocol set and other secondary endpoints were consistent with the primary endpoint, and all suggest the beneficial effect of tocilizumab compared to placebo. It is possible that the sample size of this study was too small. As discussed in Nakaoka et al., the study design was based on an estimate of tocilizumab efficacy that might have been too high. The literature review used for sample size calculation for the TAKT study reported a relapse-free rate of 83% at week 24. Even though the sample size and event calculations assumed a conservative effect size of 75% for tocilizumab compared to 25% for placebo (with a hazard ratio of 0.2075), it might have been still too optimistic since patients from the literature review studies could have received concomitant immunosuppressants. If the true hazard ratio is larger than what is assumed in the original design, the study will be underpowered. Table 4.6 shows the power of the study with 19 events at multiple values of the hazard ratio. Note that the power drops down to 72% if the true hazard ratio of tocilizumab versus placebo is 0.3 which still justifies an effective treatment.

If the option to increase the sample size/events was added to the design, the trial might have had the chance to demonstrate a statistically significant treatment benefit. To illustrate a hypothetical redesign of the TAKT study using sample size re-estimation, first consider a general two-stage design with early efficacy/futility stopping in the interim. Let Z_1 and Z_2 denote the Wald statistics in the interim and final analyses. Let (c_1, c_2) and (b_1, b_2) be the efficacy and futility boundaries for interim and final analyses which can be derived from any spending function approach such as Lan and DeMets (1983). Typically, nonbinding futility boundaries are used for confirmatory trials. To add on the option for sample size increase, the promising zone approach (Mehta and Pocock, 2011) can be applied. In this approach, interim results are categorized into a favorable, promising, and unfavorable zone in the case of no early stopping in the interim. The sample size would be increased only if the interim results fall into the promising zone which is commonly defined by conditional power. For example, if the conditional power is between 30% and 90%, the sample size would be increased to reach the target conditional power of 90%. If the conditional power is greater than 90%, interim results are considered favorable, and the trial can continue to the end until the planned sample size is reached. On the other hand, if the conditional power is less than 30%, it doesn't warrant a sample size increase since a nonrealistic large

TABLE 4.6

Study Power with 19 Events under Different Assumptions for Hazard Ratio with O'Brien Fleming Efficacy Boundary, One-Sided Alpha 0.025, Sample SIZE 34, Accrual 47 Weeks

True Hazard Ratio	Power with 19 Events	Study Duration (Week)
0.2075	90%	54
0.25	83%	52
0.3	72%	50
0.4	49%	47

sample size increase would be needed to reach adequate conditional power which might not be feasible. Denote the conditional power by:

$$CP_{z_1,\delta} = P_\delta \left(Z_2 > c_2 \mid z_1 \right)$$

where z_1 is the observed value of the Wald statistics in the interim and δ is the reference value for the hazard ratio for conditional power evaluation. Assume that there will be a flat 50% increase in sample size/events if the conditional power falls between 30% and 90%. The interim decision rule can be described as follows:

- If $Z_1 > c_1$, stop the trial early for efficacy
- If $Z_1 < b_1$, stop the trial early for futility
- If $b_1 \leq Z_1 \leq c_1$, the trial is considered falling into the continuation region where three scenarios could happen:
  - If $CP_{z_1,\delta} > 90\%$, the trial is considered falling into the favorable zone and the trial continues to the end without increasing sample size/events.
  - If $30\% \leq CP_{z_1,\delta} \leq 90\%$, the trial is considered falling into the promising zone and increasing sample size.
  - If $CP_{z_1,\delta} < 30\%$, the trial is considered falling into the unfavorable zone and the trial will continue to the end without increasing the sample size/events.

A practical rule for sample size adaption in the promising zone is to increase the sample size/events to achieve 90% conditional power subject to a cap. The cap for the sample size increase is often set to be 50%–100% for efficient design performance. The TAKT study was planned to enroll 34 subjects and collect 19 events to target a hazard ratio of 0.02075. The interim analysis was performed when 13 events were observed. With O'Brien–Fleming efficacy-spending function, the Wald scale boundaries in the interim and final look are 2.471 and 1.997, and the *p*-value scale boundaries are 0.0135 and 0.0459. In the interim, the study didn't cross the efficacy or futility boundary. With the sample size adaptation design described above, the interim results of the trial fell into the continuation region. We can evaluate whether the interim results warrant sample size/event increase using conditional power. The conditional power is given by:

$$P\left(Z_2 > 1.997 \mid z_1 \right) = 1 - \Phi \left(\frac{1.997 - \sqrt{\frac{D_1}{D}} z_1}{\sqrt{\frac{D - D_1}{D}}} + log(\delta)\sqrt{\frac{D - D_1}{4}} \right) \qquad (4.1)$$

where D_1 is the number of events observed before interim, D is the total number of events, δ is the referenced hazard ratio. The referenced hazard ratio is unknown and is often replaced by the observed estimate in the interim. Therefore, $D_1 = 13$ and $D = 19$. Table 4.7 shows a few hypothetical scenarios with the interim results. For example, if the estimated hazard ratio in the interim is 0.25 and the observed statistics is 2.2, the conditional power computed by (4.1) is 70% which warrants the increase in sample size and events. With a 50% increase in sample size and events, the conditional power is boosted to 91%.

For an adaptive design with sample size re-estimation, special statistical methods are needed to ensure that type I error rate is preserved despite a data-dependent change to the sample size. A few approaches have been developed including Cui, Hung, and Wang (1999), Lehmacher and Wassmer (1999), Chen et al. (2004), Müller and Schäfer (2001), Mehta and Pocock (2011). These approaches can be classified into three streams. The methods by Cui et al. (1999) and Lehmacher and Wassmer (1999) are based on the weighted combination test where the prefixed weights are used to combine the incremental statistics from all stages. Chen et al. (2004) showed that one can use the regular unadjusted statistics for the final test if the sample size/events are increased only when the conditional power is greater than 50%. This approach is appealing to clinicians since there is no adjustment needed to the statistics or the final test boundary even if the sample size is increased. The idea behind Müller and Schäfer (2001) is to preserve the conditional type I error rate and adjust the final test boundary but keep the statistics unadjusted. If the sample size adaptation is desired for a conditional power below 50%, one needs to either adjust the test statistics by the weighted combination test or modify the final test boundary by preserving the conditional type I error rate. The two approaches relate to each other. In fact, Mehta and Pocock (2011) and Gao et al. (2008) have shown that the two methods are equivalent at least for the two-stage design.

Although type I error rate control has been well addressed by published methods, there is limited research on the optimality of the sample size adaptation rule. Two important questions are yet to be answered: when to increase the sample size and how much to increase it. As explained previously, the idea of Mehta and Pocock (2011) is to increase the sample size in a predefined promising zone. Jennison and Turnbull (2015) developed another approach

TABLE 4.7

Interim Estimates and Corresponding Conditional Power

Observed Hazard Ratio in the Interim	Observed Z Statistics in the Interim	Conditional Power	Zone
0.27	2.36	0.94	Favorable
0.35	1.89	0.70	Promising
0.48	1.32	0.24	Unfavorable

based on maximizing the expected utility. This approach also results in a promising zone design. In this approach, a promising zone and a corresponding decision rule for a sample size increase are derived implicitly by solving an optimization problem that is characterized by an objective function and constraint. The objective function balances the trade-off between the conditional power gain and sample size increase. This design is optimal in terms of unconditional power among all the promising zone designs that have the same initial sample size, maximum sample size, and expected sample size.

Jennison and Turnbull (2015) set up a gold standard optimal design to benchmark other alternative promising zone designs. Hsiao, Liu, and Mehta (2018) present a constraint-promising zone design where the constraint is imposed to ensure a minimal conditional power. This constrained promising zone design is evaluated against the optimal unconstrained Jennison and Turnbull (2015) design and against a constrained version of the Jennison and Turnbull design. The constrained promising zone design has comparable performance to the constraint Jennison and Turnbull design. The unconstrained Jennison and Turnbull design has a slightly better unconditional power. Compared to the constrained design, the promising zone of the unconstrained Jennison and Turnbull design starts early. This means that the sample size increase could be triggered with lower conditional power. On the other hand, the constrained design only increases the sample size if adequate conditional power can be reached with the additional investment of sample size. Whether to focus on unconditional power or conditional power can be evaluated case by case.

4.3.2 Seamless Phase II/III Designs with Treatment Selection

In traditional drug development, separate trials are conducted to select among k experimental treatment arms (phase II) and confirm the efficacy of the selected treatment(s) (phase III). For generality, the k experimental arms are referred to as "treatments" in this section, though most often sponsors aim to choose among k doses of a single drug. Seamless phase II/III designs, a type of adaptive design which combines phase II and phase III objectives into a single trial, have been developed to shorten development timelines, curb costs, and reduce the burden on patients. For drug development in rare diseases, such designs are especially attractive considering the limited patient populations and high unmet needs.

Seamless phase II/III designs with interim treatment selection, often referred to as "drop-the-losers" designs (Sampson and Sill, 2005), most frequently consist of two stages. In Stage 1, n_1 subjects are randomized to each of the k experimental treatments and (usually) a control arm. At the end of this stage, one or more of the experimental treatments is selected to proceed according to a prespecified selection rule. In Stage 2, n_2 additional subjects are randomized to each selected treatment, as well as the control arm, if applicable. The final efficacy analysis typically takes the form of a hypothesis test incorporating data from both stages and is therefore considered to be inferentially seamless. Unlike some other adaptive designs, such as a multiarm multistage (MAMS) study (Wason and Jaki, 2012), seamless phase II/III designs permit prespecification of the overall sample size for the study. Operationally seamless phase II/III designs, where only Stage 2 data is used in the final analysis, are not considered in this section.

The critical challenge, as well as a key advantage, of inferentially seamless phase II/III studies is that data from Stage 1 is combined with data from Stage 2 in the final efficacy analysis. On one hand, adopting such a design for rare diseases saves sample size and recruitment time. On the other hand, since only a treatment exhibiting favorable response at Stage 1 is selected for Stage 2, a naïve final test that simply pools data from both stages is subject to selection bias that results in type 1 error inflation, and corresponding point estimates will be biased (Cohen and Sackrowitz, 1989; Tappin, 1992). The magnitude of the type 1 error rate inflation and bias increases with k and when the true responses across treatments are similar or equal (Bauer et al., 2010).

For hypothesis testing, one must account for the fact that only a subset of the treatment arms in Stage 1 was selected. One approach frequently used in the context of drop-the-losers designs is described in Posch et al. (2005), a generalization of Bauer and Kieser (1999). This closed testing procedure using p-value combination tests can be applied to a broad class of group sequential designs beyond classical seamless phase II/III designs, allowing for the possibility of stopping early for futility or adding arms in Stage 2. In the final test, the p-value based on subjects from Stage 1 is multiplicity-adjusted (for example, with the Simes procedure or, with a continuous outcome and a control arm, the Dunnett procedure) and combined with the Stage 2 p-value using a combination function (such as the weighted inverse normal or Fisher's combination function). Another family of approaches is based on a more traditional group sequential framework; one example is the optimal seamless phase II/III design for binary, quickly observable outcomes developed by Thall et al. (1988). The trial is terminated if the maximum Stage 1 test statistic across treatment arms is less than a certain threshold y_1 ; otherwise, additional patients are randomized between the selected treatment (here, the treatment with the highest test statistic) and the control in Stage 2. The final test is performed using data pooled across both stages, and the null hypothesis is rejected if this final test statistic exceeds a different threshold y_2. For specific parameters, one can directly compute optimal designs that minimize the total sample size and their corresponding thresholds y_1 and y_2. Schaid et al. (1990) extend this design to accommodate time-to-event outcomes and to allow multiple Stage 1 experimental treatments to be evaluated in Stage 2. Other group sequential approaches include Stallard and Todd (2003) and Kelly et al. (2005). A third approach, proposed by Koenig et al. (2008), is the adaptive Dunnett test procedure, based on the conditional error rate of a single-stage Dunnett test.

Methods for point and interval estimation that adjust for selection bias have also been developed for seamless phase II/III designs. Sampson and Sill (2005), in addition to originating the term "drop-the-losers" for such designs, propose an interval estimation method for normal endpoints. This approach leverages the work of Cohen and Sackrowitz (1989), who developed a uniformly minimum-variance conditionally unbiased estimator for the mean of the selected treatment under the normal distribution. Kimani et al. (2014) provide a review and comparison of multiple subsequent interval estimation methods developed for the normal case. For binary endpoints, Tappin (1992) derives the uniformly minimum-variance unbiased estimator (UMVUE) of the response rate for the selected treatment, along similar lines of argument as Cohen and Sackrowitz (1989). The UMVUE was found to exist if ties are broken based on prespecified preferences but does not exist when ties are broken randomly (Tappin, 1992). Sill and Sampson (2009) follow the conditional approach of Tappin (1992) to derive an interval estimation procedure, thereby extending their earlier work to accommodate binary endpoints. The hypothesis testing approach of Posch et al. (2005) can also be inverted to obtain confidence intervals.

In most of the literature referenced above, the seamless phase II/III designs that are explored include a control arm in both Stages 1 and 2, such that all experimental therapies are assessed against that control. However, due to high unmet medical need or difficulties with patient recruitment, a control arm may not be feasible in certain rare disease settings. Instead, the treatment effect of the experimental arms can be compared to a specified value, representing either a clinically meaningful threshold or the expected course of the disease process (based on a natural history study and/or other external data). Some hypothesis testing approaches are essentially unchanged under such a setting (Posch et al., 2005). Others require modification; for example, Thall et al. (1989) extend previous work (Thall et al., 1988) to allow for an uncontrolled Stage 1, with a control arm only appearing in Stage 2. For fully uncontrolled studies evaluating a binary endpoint, Jazić et al. (2021) propose a novel testing and interval estimation procedure based on an unconditional exact likelihood. While this exact approach provides power gains and tighter confidence intervals compared to existing methods (Posch et al., 2005; Sill and Sampson, 2009), factors influenced by small sample properties (such as the choice of n_1/n_2 and tie-breaking criteria) must be carefully considered in designing such a study.

Key early papers in the development of two-stage drop-the-losers designs assume the use of the same endpoint in Stages 1 and 2 (Thall et al., 1988; Sampson and Sill, 2005); the selection bias and associated type 1 error inflation are most salient for this case. However, in most therapeutic areas, phase III endpoints used for registration require a lengthy time horizon to demonstrate durable clinical efficacy. Phase II endpoints are typically chosen to provide a preliminary indication of clinical benefit while allowing a dose to be chosen relatively quickly. As such, methodology has been developed to handle seamless phase II/III designs where Stages 1 and 2 evaluate different but correlated endpoints (Todd and Stallard, 2005). Friede et al. (2011) propose a framework for the analysis of the Stage 2 endpoint that controls the family-wise error rate (FWER) when treatment selection is based on the Stage 1 endpoint. Stallard (2010) takes a similar approach while allowing any measurement of the Stage 2 endpoint available at the end of Stage 1 to also factor into treatment selection. Kunz et al. (2014) introduce an algorithm that chooses between the approaches of Stallard (2010) and Friede et al. (2011) depending on the estimated probability that each method correctly selects the most effective treatment, given the observed data. The resulting tests are conservative; the extent of which depends on the specific selection rule, treatment effect on the Stage 1 endpoint, and correlation between the Stage 1 and Stage 2 endpoints.

One aspect of these designs that is worth examining is the selection rule after Stage 1. Much of the literature assumes that treatment with the highest point estimate on the Stage 1 endpoint proceeds to Stage 2 (Stallard and Todd, 2003; Thall et al., 1988; Kimani et al., 2014), and this assumption underlies the point and interval estimation methods discussed previously. For binary outcomes, these rules include prespecified treatment selection preferences in the case of ties; particularly in the rare disease setting, the chance of ties among treatment arms is nontrivial (Sill and Sampson, 2009). Such rigid selection rules may be risky when the endpoints used in Stages 1 and 2 differ; indeed, the relationship between such endpoints often is not fully characterized. Friede et al. (2011) recommend that, if the Stage 1 endpoint is not a validated surrogate for the Stage 2 endpoint, multiple treatments should be permitted to continue if they all perform similarly on the Stage 1 endpoint and demonstrate benefit over the control arm. For some testing approaches, including Posch et al. (2005), the FWER is still controlled even if the selection rule is violated; however, point and interval estimators constructed around specific selection rules may perform more poorly (Jazić et al., 2021).

However, there are many other options for selection rules. For example, Stage 1 response rates can inform Bayesian posterior probabilities that can be used to drop less efficacious treatment arms (Inoue et al., 2002; Berry et al., 2010). Instead of dropping arms altogether, response-adaptive randomization can be used to update the randomization ratio in favor of more efficacious arms—both frequentist (Zhu et al., 2020; Zhan et al., 2021; Cui et al., 2021) and Bayesian approaches (Wason and Trippa, 2014; Yap and Cheung, 2018) have been developed for seamless phase II/III trials. In practice, the decision of which experimental treatment(s) proceed to Stage 2 is based on the totality of the evidence, including safety considerations as well as efficacy (Barnes et al., 2010; Chen et al., 2014).

There have been more recent extensions to seamless phase II/III designs in the literature. When the endpoints used in Stages 1 and 2 differ, Stage 1 subjects assigned to a treatment that is not selected are typically not followed up for the measurement of the Stage 2 endpoint and are not included in the final test. In some settings, such as rare diseases where the disease course may be poorly understood and historical data may be sparse, sponsors may wish to measure the Stage 2 endpoint on these subjects to better characterize the disease process and use a potentially more efficient multiplicity adjustment procedure (Friede et al., 2011; Quan et al., 2018). Bowden and Glimm (2014) and Wason et al. (2017) generalize the drop-the-losers design to incorporate multiple stages. Quan et al. (2020) propose a seamless phase II/III/IIIb design, in which each stage evaluates a different endpoint (where Stage 2 is used for accelerated approval and Stage 3 is used for final approval). The design and analysis of seamless phase II/III studies with treatment selection clearly remain an active area of methodological research.

4.3.3 Master Protocol Designs

A challenge in rare diseases is the limited size of the patient population which is often not feasible for a traditional large confirmation trial. Not surprisingly, recent years have seen more and more research and applications in master protocol design, including Umbrella, Basket, and Platform trials, in rare diseases. For example, in oncology, it is not uncommon to combine multiple rare diseases as defined by a common biomarker signature in one trial to provide confirmatory evidence.

Woodcock and LaVange (2017) argued that the precision medicine approach to developing targeted therapies requires addressing multiple questions involving different diseases or molecular/genotype subgroups in the same disease. These questions cannot be answered efficiently by conducting conventional independent trials. Woodcock and LaVange (2017) pointed out that a solution to solving these challenges more efficiently is a master protocol (such as basket designs), i.e., one overarching protocol designed to answer multiple questions. FDA (2018) published a draft guidance for developing oncology drugs and biologics using master protocols, further opening the door of a regulatory pathway to develop a targeted therapy for multiple rare or ultrarare diseases or diseases with low-frequency molecular or genotype subgroups (niche indications), where study eligibility is based on criteria other than the traditional disease definition (Woodcock and LaVange, 2017).

Typical trials adopted in master protocols include Umbrella, Basket, and Platform trials. Umbrella trial studies multiple targeted therapies in the context of a single disease and the Platform trial is a subtype of an Umbrella trial allowing therapies to enter or leave the trial continuously. A Basket trial studies a single-targeted therapy in the context of multiple diseases or disease subtypes. The following sections provide an overview of these trial designs as well as examples for illustrations.

4.3.3.1 Umbrella/Platform Trials

There are three types of Umbrella designs. The first is called the MAMS design (Follmann et al., 1994; Wason and Jaki, 2012; Wason and Trippa, 2014). It is considered a special case of the group sequential design, in which multiple arms are included in multiple stages, and each arm can be allowed to stop early due to futility.

The second type of Umbrella design is called drop-the-loser design (Wason et al., 2017) or select-the-winner design. Similar to the MAMS design, at each interim analysis, a prespecified number of arms with the best performance and the control arm are allowed to enter the next stage. The details of this design can be found in Section 4.3.2.

The third type of Umbrella design is called adaptive randomization (also see Section 4.3.2). At each interim look, the randomization ratio for each arm will be updated and determined by accumulated data. The statistical method, usually Bayesian, in calculating the adaptive randomization ratio needs to be prespecified and then be used to dynamically adjust the randomization ratio in favor of better drugs according to the accumulated study data.

When an Umbrella trial of either above-mentioned type allows compounds to leave and enter the trial continuously, it becomes a Platform trial. Below is an example of a Platform trial adopting Bayesian adaptive randomization.

4.3.3.1.1 I-SPY2 Trial

The I-SPY program contains a series of umbrella/platform trials to examine treatments for breast cancer, at the heart of which is the ground-breaking I-SPY2 platform trial for neoadjuvant treatment of locally advanced breast cancer. The I-SPY2 (Barker et al., 2009) is a phase II study that simultaneously evaluated multiple drugs from different sponsors featuring Bayesian adaptive randomization. It is designed in an adaptive fashion to allow up to five agents (or combinations of agents) to be evaluated at the same time. New patients with a specific molecular subtype are assigned to agents or combinations showing higher response rates within that subtype allowing for a more rapid evaluation. Stop for success is allowed in the experimental group when the Bayesian predictive probability of success reaches a prespecified threshold (usually 85%) for any molecular subtype. When that occurs, the agent or combination is graduated from the trial. Stopping for futility is recommended to an agent or combination if the probability falls below 10% for all biomarker signatures and it is then dropped from the trial. New agents can be added to the trial at any time as the testing agents are either graduated or dropped.

Up to now, there were about 1,600 patients enrolled in this study, and 16 agents completed evaluations, resulting in three approved drugs (accelerated approvals). To learn more details on each substudy and agent, please go to the website of https://www.ispytrials.org, which also provides a list of publications reporting the study results.

Another example is the STAMPEDE Trial, a Platform Umbrella trial adopting the design type of MAMS, on prostate cancer. More details can be found on www.stampedetrial.org.

4.3.3.2 Basket Trial

Basket trial studies a single therapy targeting multiple diseases or disease subtypes. These diseases or disease subtypes are called baskets. When multiple rare diseases can be defined by a common biomarker signature or a disease has multiple disease subtypes of low frequency, a Basket trial is useful to provide mutually supportive evidence for these diseases or subtypes (baskets) as a combined group (Cunanan et al., 2017).

Oncology therapy development is the area where Basket trials have gained the most popularity due to the shift of oncology research from conventional cytotoxic therapy to personalized therapies that target specific genetic or molecular aberrations. In a Basket trial, patients with cancers of various types of tumor histology that harbor specific molecular aberrations are recruited in the same trial. One investigational therapy is tested in multiple patient populations of different tumor histology with the objective of selecting the basket(s) that show promising responses to the investigational therapy.

By studying multiple diseases in one study, Basket trials can provide advantages such as higher operational efficiency and increased probability of success compared to traditional trials and can consequently shorten the time of drug development.

Recently, advances in identifying molecular aberrations in disease pathways via Basket trials go beyond oncology. In 2018, FDA published the guidance for the industry for developing targeted therapies in low-frequency molecular subsets of a disease (FDA, 2018). Target therapies are defined as drugs or therapeutic biological products intended for populations that are subsets of clinically defined diseases and are identified using diagnostic testing. In this guidance, FDA states that they will accept grouping patients with different molecular alterations if it is reasonable to expect that the grouped patients will have similar pharmacological responses based on a strong scientific rationale, which can be computational (e.g., in silico), experimental (e.g., in vitro or animal experiments), or clinical evidence. FDA also gives recommendations on how to group patients with different molecular alterations for eligibility in clinical trials. It describes the general approaches to evaluating the benefits and risks of targeted therapies within a clinically defined disease where some molecular alterations may occur at low frequencies.

To analyze the data generated in the Basket trials, there are different approaches on the level of information borrowing between different baskets. Below is a summary of these methods and corresponding examples.

4.3.3.2.1 No Borrowing

The first category is to ignore similarities among baskets by analyzing individual basket independently, without borrowing information across baskets. This type of design can be used for screening subtypes that are responsive to the therapy by utilizing a common screening platform. However, if certain baskets have similar responses to the drug, not borrowing information across these baskets loses the opportunity of increased power or saving sample sizes in these baskets, consequently leading to a delay in developing novel medicines.

BRAF V600 Study (Hyman et al. 2015) was a histology-independent phase II, open-label, basket study to assess the efficacy and safety of vemurafenib in participants with BRAF V600 mutation-positive nonmelanoma cancers. Patients were enrolled in six prespecified baskets (also called cohorts in this example) (non-small-cell lung cancer, ovarian cancer, colorectal cancer, cholangiocarcinoma, breast cancer, and multiple myeloma), as well as a seventh (all-others) cohort for any other BRAF V600 mutation-positive cancer. Due to the challenge in recruiting patients in the cohort of breast cancer, two cohorts were added in the middle of the study: patients with Erdheim–Chester disease (ECD) or Langerhans' cell histiocytosis (LCH) and those with anaplastic thyroid cancer. Patients in all cohorts received vemurafenib except in the cohort of colorectal cancer patients were randomized to receive vemurafenib monotherapy and vemurafenib+cetuximab due to data from the phase I study indicated that vemurafenib alone had insufficient activity in BRAF V600-mutated colorectal cancer patients.

The primary endpoint was the objective response rate at week 8. Simon's two-stage design (Simon, 1989) was used for each disease-specific basket to minimize the number of patients treated if vemurafenib was deemed ineffective. The enrollment target was calibrated to control the two-sided type I error rate at 0.1 at the ineffective response rate of 15% and have 80% power at a high response rate of 45% for the primary efficacy endpoint. A response rate of 35% would be considered low but promising and indicative of efficacy. The basket named all-others was purely exploratory with no inferential methods planned.

A total of 122 patients were enrolled, 95 were treated with vemurafenib monotherapy and 27 with vemurafenib+cetuximab. Among different cohorts, the ECD/LCH cohort included 22 patients with ECD; of whom 12 (55%) responded to the treatment with a durable response (Diamond et al 2016). Data from this trial led to the FDA's approval of vemurafenib for the treatment of BRAF V600 mutation-positive ECD. This study established an example of a basket trial with no information borrowing.

4.3.3.2.2 Complete Borrowing

The second category is the pool-all-baskets approach, i.e., complete borrowing of information. This approach assumes that all baskets in the trial have similar pharmacological responses to the drug, which needs to be justified by a strong scientific rationale (FDA, 2018).

Vitrakvi was granted accelerated approval for treating pediatric and adult patients with locally advanced or metastatic solid tumors harboring a neurotropic tyrosine kinase receptor (NTRK) gene fusion. The approval was primarily based on the Vitrakvi study, a basket trial utilizing the complete borrowing approach. The study pooled results from three single-arm open-label clinical trials with a total of 55 patients from 12 solid tumor types harboring the NTRK gene fusion. The efficacy was evaluated by overall response rate and duration of response. The efficacy results overall and by tumor type can be found in the Vitrakvi label (https://www.accessdata.fda.gov/drug-satfda_docs/label/2018/211710s000lbl.pdf).

The unique feature of this study is that the single arm in each of the three trials consisted of patients in multiple types of tumors or multiple baskets. It set up a precedent of regulatory approval of a therapy based on a prespecified enrollment criterion of a genetic mutation, regardless of primary tumor site of origin and histology, or the number of patients by which various solid tumor types were represented in the clinical trial. As many solid tumors of different tumor sites are rare or ultrarare diseases, separate trials for each tumor type would be infeasible. Using a Basket trial to include all tumor types harboring the NTRK gene fusion, operational and statistical efficiencies had been achieved.

4.3.3.2.3 Adaptive Borrowing

The third category is to borrow information adaptively based on the similarity of response to treatment across baskets.

4.3.3.2.4 Simon's Bayesian Design

A Bayesian adaptive method proposed by Simon et al. (2016) uses the posterior probability of homogeneity to control the amount of information borrowed at each interim look. Early stopping of enrollment of individual subgroups for either futility or strong efficacy is possible based on the interim results. By allowing multiple interim looks besides potential information borrowing between multiple subgroups, the Simon's Bayesian design is an improvement over traditional Simon's two-stage design, which allows one interim look and works for only one cohort.

At the design stage, the response rate π_k of each basket (k) to the investigational treatment is assumed to be either p_1 (representing a desirable response rate) or p_0 (representing the null response rate). In each interim analysis, the posterior probability of treatment effects being equal among strata, π, will be updated. And, subsequently, the posterior probability of the treatment being effective for a specific basket k [$Pr(\pi_k = p_1 \mid \text{data})$] will also be updated, where $Pr(\pi_k = p_1 \mid \text{data})$ is the weighted average of the posterior probability of treatment being active overall under complete borrowing assuming homogeneous π_ks, and of the kth stratum being active under no borrowing assuming π_ks are independent, using π as the weight. In the end, $Pr(\pi_k = p_1 \mid \text{data})$ will then be evaluated against the decision rules to determine which baskets will be terminated and which will continue accrual.

4.3.3.2.5 Chen et al.'s Design Combining No-Borrowing and Complete-Borrowing

Chen et al. (2016) proposed a design that combines the approaches of no-borrowing and complete-borrowing in one study to enable the application of Basket trial design in confirmatory studies by controlling type I error rates. It allows for an interim analysis in which the responses of an individual basket are evaluated independently against a predefined decision criterion α_t for potential pruning. When the *p*-value of a basket is greater than α_t, it will be pruned; otherwise, it will go to the second stage. Therefore, there is no borrowing across baskets at the interim look. The remaining baskets are pooled and evaluated at level α^* for the final analysis, where α^* is derived so that the overall type I error rate under the global null hypothesis is well controlled.

Let Y_{i1} be the standardized test statistics based on the endpoint used for pruning at the interim analysis and Y_{i2} be the standardized test statistics based on the endpoint for pooling for the *i*-th tumor indication at the final analysis ($i = 1, \ldots, k$). Let $Q_0(\alpha^* \mid \alpha_t, m) = \mathrm{Pr}_{H_0}(\{Y_{i1} > Z_{1-\alpha_t} \text{ for } i = 1, \ldots, m\}, V_m > Z_{1-\alpha}^*)(1-\alpha_t)^{(k-m)}$ be the probability of the *m* baskets entering the second stage and *Vm* being statistically significant at the α^* level, where *m* is the total number of baskets in the final analysis, V_m is the sum of Y_{i2} ($i = 1, \ldots, m$) divided by $\sqrt{m}$. Then, the adjusted type I error rate α^* can be obtained from the equation

$$\sum_{m=1}^{k} c(k,m) Q_0(\alpha^* \mid \alpha_t, m) = \alpha,$$ where $c(k, m)$ is the number of choices for selecting *m* baskets from *k*. The R code can be found in Chen et al (2016).

4.3.3.2.6 Adaptive Borrowing through Bayesian-Structured Framework

Information borrowing can be more flexible and adaptive, driven by the results at the interim looks using a more structured Bayesian framework. Consider designing a basket trial with *K* baskets, and assume θ_k the treatment effect for the *k*th basket. If we model the $\theta_k's$ with independent normal distributions, with non-informative priors, $\theta_k \sim N\left(\rho_k, \omega^2\right)$, $k = 1, \ldots, K$, where $\rho_k's$ and ω^2 are hyperparameters, then there is no borrowing across the groups. Wathen et al. (2008) proposed a Bayesian method that assumes independent normal distributions for $\theta_k's$ and allows borrowing historical information on the treatment effect from the SOC.

The full Bayesian hierarchical model (BHM) proposed by Thall et al. (2003) and Berry et al. (2013) models $\theta_k \sim N\left(m, \sigma^2\right)$, $k = 1, \ldots, K$, and the second level of distributions on m : $m \sim N\left(m_0, \sigma_0^2\right)$, and σ^2: $\sigma^2 \sim$ Inverse Gamma (a, b) to allow borrowing between baskets. A small value of σ^2 induces strong information borrowing across baskets, whereas a large value of σ^2 indicates little information borrowing. Thus, the degree of information borrowing is controlled by σ^2, which is jointly estimated with other model parameters.

Based on the same framework, the calibrated Bayesian hierarchical model (CBHM) proposed by Chu and Yuan (2018) suggested to estimate the variance σ^2 through a monotone increasing function of a similarity measure of the treatment effects across baskets. For binary endpoint, the chi-square test statistic of homogeneity (denoted by *T*) can be used as the measure of similarity of the treatment effect across baskets. The function is calibrated using simulation so that information is strongly borrowed across baskets if their treatment effects are similar and barely borrowed if the treatment effects are heterogeneous. In Chu and Yuan (2018), an exponential function was used $\sigma^2 = \exp\{a + b^* \log(T)\}$, where a and b are tuning parameters that characterize the relationship between σ^2 and T, to satisfy given type I and type II error rates. Based on simulations, they showed that the CBHM approach controls the type I error rate better than the BHM approach.

The four different approaches of adaptive borrowing have different features, but all include interim analysis to allow early decisions (Table 4.8). Unfortunately, regulatory approvals based on clinical trials adopting these designs could not be found to the best of our knowledge.

TABLE 4.8

Characteristics of the Statistical Methods for Basket Trial Designs

Characteristic		Simon's Two-Stage Design[a]	Simon's Bayesian Design	Wathen's STI Design	Chen et al. Design
Design	Applicable in phase II trials	X	X	X	
	Applicable in phase III trials				X
	Borrowing information across subgroups		X	X	X
	Borrowing historical information			X	
	Allowing between-subgroup treatment differences	X	X	X	X
Interim Analysis	Allowing more than one interim		X	X	
	Allowing only one interim	X			X
	Early stopping for efficacy		X		
	Early stopping for futility	X	X	X	X
	Subgroup-specific stopping rule	X	X	X	X
Statistical Consideration	Continuous endpoint			X	X
	Binary endpoint	X	X	X	X
	Time-to-event endpoint			X	X
	Subgroup-level type I error rate control	X			
	Subgroup-level power target	X		X	
	Type I error rate control for global null				X
Software	Publicly available software	X	X		X

[a] The characteristics of Simon's two-stage design are evaluated under the assumption that trials for subgroups are designed and analyzed separately.

4.3.4 Crossover Design

The double-blind randomized controlled trial (RCT) has been considered the gold standard for assessing the safety and efficacy of investigational new drugs. These trials are very effective at overcoming bias and yielding high-quality evidence because subjects are allocated at random to receive either the study drug or a comparator treatment/placebo and the subjects are unaware of their assigned treatment group. Regulatory guidance requests that drugs for rare diseases are assessed according to the same rules as established for common diseases (EMA/CHMP, 2006).

At the same time, challenges in conducting standard parallel-group RCTs in rare diseases are well documented. Some alternative clinical trial designs have focused on allowing subjects to receive more than one treatment. The most common example of such a design is the crossover design. In a crossover trial, subjects are given predefined sequences of treatments, and the objective is to study the differences between the individual treatments. Each treatment period lasts for the same amount of time, and there may be a washout period between treatment periods where the subjects receive no treatment. As each subject acts as the subject's own control, the obvious advantage of a crossover design is that it allows consideration of within-subject variability in responses to treatments. Since several observations are made on each subject, another advantage is that fewer subjects are required than in an equivalently powered parallel group design.

Along with the advantages, there are some disadvantages as well to the crossover trial (Senn, 2002):

1. There are many conditions or indications for which crossover trials would not be appropriate. For example, acute conditions for which there is a reasonable probability that the subject might be cured after treatment. It is only appropriate to use a crossover design for experiments where the condition to be treated is chronic and relatively stable. The treatment must result in a reversible outcome, and participants must return to their pretreatment condition soon after treatment stops. This may not be an issue for rare diseases because many rare diseases are chronic conditions that progress over time.

2. Treatment differences in one period might be different from those in later periods due to treatment by period interaction. One cause of this is carryover, i.e., the persistence of the effect of the treatment given in a period in subsequent treatment periods. In other words, if a subject receives treatment A during the first period and treatment B during the second period, then measurements taken during the second period could be a result of the direct effect of treatment B administered during the second period and/or the carryover or residual effect of treatment A administered during the first period. The

treatment received in earlier periods becomes a confounding factor for later periods and therefore we cannot justify the comparative treatment difference between individual treatments without the possibility of biased estimates. The incorporation of washout periods in the experimental design can diminish the impact of carryover effects. A washout period is defined as the intervening time between treatment periods to allow the drug from the preceding period to be washed out of the subject's system. The length of the washout period usually is determined as some multiples of the half-life of the pharmaceutical product within the population of interest. Additional considerations beyond half-life may be given in cases where the treatment effect from the previous period is expected to last for a longer duration and therefore the washout period would be longer. If there are constraints on the length of the washout period, it could be enhanced by only considering later time points in the treatment period (when carryover is unlikely to be present) in the endpoint definition. Note that it is not the presence of carryover effects per se that leads to treatment effect comparisons being biased, but rather the presence of differential carryover effects, i.e., the carryover effect due to treatment A differs from the carryover effect due to treatment B.

3. Crossover trials may cause inconvenience to subjects and consequently have higher dropouts. This is because the subjects are required to receive more than one treatment and the total duration of follow-up will be longer than in an equivalent parallel group design. However, sometimes subjects may be interested in the opportunity to receive different types of treatment. The opportunity for every subject to receiving active treatment will also enhance the recruitment and retention efforts which are especially critical for clinical trials on rare diseases.

The following subsections introduce different types of crossover designs.

4.3.4.1 AB/BA Design

The simplest and one of the most used crossover designs is the AB/BA crossover or two-treatment, two-period (2×2) crossover. In a typical case, subjects are randomly assigned in a 1:1 ratio to either receive treatment A followed by the washout period followed by treatment B or treatment B followed by the washout period followed by treatment A.

4.3.4.1.1 Notation and Model for the AB/BA Design

We will denote by t, p, and s, respectively, the number of treatments, periods, and sequences. So, for the AB/BA crossover, we have $t = 2$, $p = 2$, and $s = 2$. The response for a given subject within a given period is represented by a linear combination of treatment and period effect.

For a continuous outcome, the statistical model can be represented by a linear model (Jones and Kenward, 2014):

$$Y_{ijk} = \mu + \pi_j + \tau_{d(i,j)} + s_{ik} + e_{ijk} \qquad (4.2)$$

where

Y_{ijk} : response observed on kth subject in period j of sequence i;

μ : overall mean;

π_j : effect of period j, $j = 1...p$;

$\tau_{d(i,j)}$: effect of treatment corresponding to period j of sequence i, $d(i,j) = 1..t$;

s_{ik} : effect of kth subject on sequence i, $i=1..s$, $k = 1...ni$;

e_{ijk} : random error term with zero mean and variance σ^2;

The subject effect can be assumed to be an unknown fixed parameter or could be assumed as a random variable with zero mean and variance σ_s^2. If the subject effect is assumed as fixed, then the analysis will use information from within-subject comparison only. However, in certain cases, the subject totals can be used to provide indirect treatment comparisons or subjects have dropped out and partial data from subjects needs to be used, it may be advantageous to assume subject effects as random. If the carryover effect needs to be included in the model, the term $\lambda_{d(i,j-1)}$ could be added to the model. The term $\lambda_{d(i,j-1)}$ represents the carryover effect of treatment $d(i, j-1)$ and is equal to 0 for $j = 1$.

In crossover trials, the main objective usually is to conduct estimation and inference related to the true difference between the treatment groups. The assumption of no carryover effect is made; under this assumption, an unbiased estimate of treatment differences can be obtained. The recommendation is to design the trial with the best knowledge of adequate washout period and acknowledge that the treatment difference estimate is conditional on the assumption of no carryover effect (Hilgers et al., 2016).

Consider the statistical model (4.2) for AB/BA crossover design along with normal distribution for the error term and random subject effect. If we define $d_{1k} = Y_{11k} - Y_{12k}$ and $d_{2k} = Y_{21k} - Y_{22k}$ as period differences, then an unbiased estimate of treatment difference can be obtained as:

$$E\left(\frac{\bar{d}_{1.} - \bar{d}_{2.}}{2} \right) = \tau_1 - \tau_2$$

Assuming that the sample size allocation is equal for the two sequences, $n_1 = n_2 = n/2$, and the within sequence variances $S_{d1.}^2 = S_{d2.}^2 = S_d^2$ are the same, then the mean difference, $(\bar{d}_{1.} - \bar{d}_{2.})/2$, has the variance $S_d^2 (1/n_1 + 1/n_2)/4 = S_d^2/n$.

The null hypothesis $\tau_1 = \tau_2$ can be tested using the test statistic:

$$T = \frac{\left(\dfrac{\bar{d}_{1.} - \bar{d}_{2.}}{2}\right)}{\sqrt{\dfrac{S_d^2}{n}}}$$

which has a Student's t-distribution with $n-2$ degrees of freedom. The analysis can be readily implemented using existing statistical software, e.g., SAS procedure PROC MIXED.

4.3.4.1.2 Sample Size for AB/BA Design

If we assume that the observations are normally distributed and the sample size for each sequence is n/2 and the within-subject variance is σ^2, the sample size can be calculated using:

$$n = \frac{2\sigma^2 \left(Z_{1-\alpha/2} + Z_{1-\beta}\right)^2}{\delta^2}$$

where $Z_{1-\alpha/2}$ and $Z_{1-\beta}$ are percentiles from standard normal distribution corresponding to type I error rate α and type II error rate β And δ is the value of the desired treatment difference. To adjust for the approximation to t distribution, the term $\frac{1}{2}Z_{1-\alpha/2}^2$ could be added to n (Guenther, 1981). For the rare disease setting, special strategies may need to be implemented to increase power (Kempf, 2018) with a smaller sample size. One strategy could be to incorporate steps for variance reduction such as taking multiple measurements at the visit and using the average as the value at the visit, use a central reader, and adjust for baseline covariates (baseline adjustment is discussed in the next paragraph). Another strategy could be to plan interim looks for safety, futility, and early evidence of efficacy, for example, via group sequential approaches. The group sequential design is discussed in Section 4.3.1, and details of analysis of group sequential AB/BA design with normally distributed endpoint are discussed in Jennison and Turnbull (2000). If the available number of subjects is small and it cannot be determined that the distribution of the outcome is approximately normal or there is presence of outlying values, nonparametric analytical approaches like permutation test which does not use normal distribution assumption would be more appropriate to construct the p value (Korn et al., 2013; Tudor and Koch, 1994). In this approach, a test statistic based on the observed values of within subject difference of first and second period or rank transformed values of such difference is computed on the observed data and then on each of the datasets formed by permuting the treatment sequence labels in all possible ways. The permutation p value is the proportion of all permuted datasets (including the original observed dataset with no permutation) that have values of the test statistic equivalent to or more extreme than the test statistic obtained using the observed data (Korn et al., 2013). The corresponding power could be assessed using simulation and may potentially be more powerful than the t-test.

4.3.4.1.3 Baseline Measurements

It is quite common to have baseline measurements in crossover trials. In the AB/BA crossover trial, we can consider baseline measurements prior to the start of the first treatment (also called study baseline) and measurements during the washout period (also called period baseline). The baseline measurements after washout could still be impacted by carryover. Therefore, only the measurement taken prior to the first treatment can be considered unambiguously a true baseline. The statistical power of crossover trials may be maximized by incorporating the baseline measurements. Several methods for the analysis of crossover trials with baseline measurements have been discussed in the literature (Mehrotra, 2014). The methods include those which ignore baseline measurements, use change from baseline as a dependent variable, use analysis of covariance with a single baseline or linear combination of baseline as a covariate, and jointly model baseline and post-baseline measurements. The literature emphasizes the importance of the variance–covariance matrix of the vector of within-subject responses in determining how incorporating baselines into the analysis can improve the precision of the treatment estimate. Under the assumption of no carryover effect, Mehrotra (2014) examined ten different approaches to incorporate baseline for the AB/BA crossover design for different variance–covariance structures and sample sizes; the final recommendation based on type I error rate and power properties was to use the difference between the two baselines as a covariate in ANCOVA. The evaluation was based on a total sample size of as low as 16 subjects and therefore relevant for clinical trials in rare diseases. The same approach has been recommended in another publication with the requirement that the washout period is at least as long as the treatment period (Senn, 2002).

4.3.4.1.4 AB/BA Design with Non-Normal Outcomes

In the previous section, we considered trials where the response variable was considered normally distributed. However, for clinical trials in rare diseases, it is relatively common that the outcomes are not even approximately normally distributed. In addition, techniques like transformation cannot be used such that standard statistical models could be applied to the transformed data.

Binary Outcomes

Several methods have been proposed for binary outcomes. Suppose that the joint outcomes for (Y_{11k}, Y_{12k}) are (00), (10), (01), and (11) where the binary indicator Y_{ijk} corresponds to the outcome from kth subject in jth period and ith sequence.

McNemar's test: One of the simplest approaches considers only the discordant outcomes (01) and (10) relative to the two treatments and assumes no period effect as well as no carryover effect. Under the null hypothesis of no direct treatment effect, the number of subjects who show a preference for a given treatment has a binomial distribution with the probability of one-half conditioned on the total number of subjects who showed a preference. The exact p value can be obtained from the binomial distribution. This is known as McNemar's test (Agresti, 2013).

Mainland–Gart test: A limitation of McNemar's test is the assumption of no period effect. Mainland–Gart test also considers the discordant joint outcomes but allows for a period effect (Gart, 1969). In addition, it is assumed that there is no carryover effect and conditional independence holds (i.e., within a given subject, responses for the two periods are independent). The test for treatment given the period effect is equivalent to Fisher's exact test for the two-by-two table in which the rows are the two sequences and the columns are the (01) and (10) discordant outcomes in McNemar's test (Gart, 1969). A large sample approximation using chi-square distribution is available for both these tests. Conditional logistic regression is another way of conducting the Mainland–Gart test (Jones and Kenward, 2014; Stokes et al., 2012). In this case, we are using the familiar logistic regression approach by conditioning on subject effects and obtaining tests and CI for direct treatment effects and other effects of interest; for small samples, it is also possible to construct a conditional exact analysis.

Prescott test: Prescott proposed an alternative to the Mainland–Gart test which includes data from subjects who show no preference (Prescott, 1981). In this case, a scoring profile of +1, 0, and −1 is created for the joint outcomes (10), (00), and (11) combined, and (01), respectively. The mean profile between the two sequences is compared using an exact trend test for the 2 (sequence) by 3 (score) contingency table.

Prescott test is the most powerful when compared to McNemar's test and Mainland–Gart test (Prescott, 1981). But the Prescott test does not provide an estimate of the treatment effect. Using a mixed model approach similar to that for continuous endpoints will allow recovery of between subject information (for applicable designs), incorporate data from subjects with incomplete data, and obtain a meaningful estimate of treatment effect and therefore should be the preferred option (Brown and Prescott, 2006) provided the sample size is not too small. This can be implemented using a generalized linear mixed model or generalized estimating equations method.

Other Types of Outcomes

The ordinal response could be analyzed using the proportional odds model (Jones and Kenward, 2014). For count data, Poisson log-linear model or its negative binomial distribution analogue as well as the generalized linear mixed model (Stroup, 2012) could be used. Analysis of time-to-event outcomes using generalization of the Wilcoxon-Mann-Whitney has been discussed (Tudor and Koch, 1994; Feingold and Gillespie, 1996).

4.3.4.2 Optimal Design for Two Treatments

In the AB/BA crossover design, the carryover effect, the treatment by period interaction, and sequence effects are all confounded or aliased with each other. This is because in the AB/BA crossover we have only three degrees of freedom between the means, one of which is for the difference in period effect and one is for the difference in treatment effect (Jones and Kenward, 2014). There is only one remaining degree of freedom for other effects if they are of interest. The sequence effect and treatment by period interaction are unlikely in a well-planned trial. However, the carryover effect could be of interest. To address this issue, alternate designs have been proposed with either more periods or more sequences. Several optimal designs have been proposed in the literature. These designs satisfy the criteria of giving minimum variance unbiased estimates for both treatment and carryover effect. One of the optimal designs with two treatments and two periods is the Balaam's design. In this design, we have four sequences AA, BB, AB, and BA (Chow and Liu, 2008). Such designs in which estimates of treatment and carryover effect are both of interest may be less applicable for rare disease clinical trials and will not be discussed further in this chapter. The recommendation is reiterated to design the trial so that the assumption of no carryover effect can be defended.

4.3.4.3 Complete Block Designs for Three or More Treatments

Unlike the case of crossover trials for two treatments, there are additional considerations when selecting the trial design for three or more treatments. To choose the most appropriate design, consideration should be given to the precision of the treatment comparisons and whether they are equally important, the number of periods that is feasible, and also the sample size (Jones and Kenward, 2014). In this section, we will focus on designs for which the number of periods is equal to the number of treatments and each subject receives each treatment only once. Usually, the intent is to select the design so that all the direct treatment differences are estimated with the same precision. Such designs are referred to as variance-balanced designs. A variance-balanced design can be easily constructed using Latin squares. A Latin square of order n is an arrangement of n symbols in a $n \times n$ square array in such a way that each symbol occurs once in each row and once in each column. In the case of crossover design, it means that each subject will receive each treatment and each treatment will occur in a period the same number of times. A Latin square design for three treatments (A, B, and C) may be represented as follows (Jones and Kenward, 2014):

	Period		
Sequence	1	2	3
1	A	B	C
2	B	C	A
3	C	A	B

The Latin square presented above is not the only one available. The alternative design could be constructed with (ACB), (BAC), and (CBA) as the three sequences.

In the absence of the carryover effect, the Latin square design is optimal in terms of the minimum variance for the comparison between any two treatment groups. For the clinical trial design, we could select one or two of the possible Latin squares at random. To achieve maximum efficiency in the presence of a simple carryover effect, the design must in addition be balanced. In a balanced design, (1) each treatment appears the same number of times in each period; (2) each subject receives each treatment exactly once; and (3) each treatment precedes every other treatment the same number of times. The design proposed so far does not satisfy this condition. Williams (1949) showed that balance can be achieved by using a specific Latin square when the number of treatments is even and using two specific Latin squares when the number of treatments is odd. An easy-to-follow algorithm for constructing William's design is available (Sheehe and Bross, 1961). For the case of three treatments, William's design consists of combining the two Latin squares presented earlier in this section. The advantage of William's design against other alternatives for a balanced design is that it requires fewer subjects for the same level of efficiency. The resulting data can be analyzed using approaches similar to what was described for the AB/BA design (e.g., linear mixed model and generalized linear mixed model). Due to more than two treatments and the resulting likelihood of type I error rate inflation from multiple comparisons, it is critical to identify a good testing strategy with a strong FWER control and adequate power in the small sample setting.

4.3.4.4 Incomplete Block Designs

In Section 4.3.4.3, we discussed crossover trial designs in which each subject received each treatment once. However, such a design may not always be practical, especially so in rare diseases. Since the subject is expected to receive all the treatments, the likelihood of dropout and therefore missing data from later periods increases. In addition, the potentially long total duration of the trial for the subject increases the likelihood of treatment by period interaction. It may also not be ethical to keep the subjects in the trial for a long duration. Therefore, it is sometimes desirable to have an incomplete block design in which subjects receive subsets of the total treatments in the trial (Senn, 2002). When all the treatment comparisons are equally important, then the treatment combinations within a subject should be balanced, i.e., the number of times a pair of treatments occurs together over the whole design should be equal for all treatment pairs. This can be achieved by constructing a balanced incomplete block (BIB) design. In a BIB design, each treatment occurs the same number of times and each pair of treatment occurs together the same number of times λ, where λ is an integer.

In the BIB design, there are "t" treatments, "s" blocks, "p" $<t$ treatments in each block, "r" occurrences of each treatment in the experiment. An expression for λ in terms of t, p, and r is as follows:

$$\lambda = \frac{r(p-1)}{(t-1)}$$

Since λ is an integer, the BIB design is not available for all combinations of t, p, and r. A BIB design for three treatments A, B, C, and block size of 2 involves blocks (AB), (AC), (BC); in this case, $\lambda = 1$. To build a crossover design with balance, we will need to treat each block as a crossover with two treatments. The BIB crossover design for three treatments and two periods is represented as follows:

	Period	
Sequence	1	2
1	A	B
2	B	A
3	A	C
4	C	A
5	B	C
6	C	B

Similarly, a BIB design for four treatments A, B, C, D, and block size of 3 involves blocks (ABC), (ABD), (ACD), (BCD); in this case $\lambda = 2$.

The model to analyze the data from BIB crossover design is similar to that described earlier. For the continuous endpoint case, we had considered the model described in (4.2). Consider the analysis of data from the BIB crossover design for three treatments and two periods. The design is a combination of three separate crossover—AB/BA, AC/CA, and BC/CB. If we consider the subject effects s_{ik} as a fixed effect, we will obtain within subject estimates of treatment difference. There is, however, another level of information on treatment difference which is available from subject totals. For example, we can obtain an estimate of difference between treatment A and treatment B from sequences 1 and 2; this would be the within-subject information. If we consider the total from periods 1 and 2 for sequences 3, 4, 5, and 6 and consider their difference, we will obtain another estimate of the difference between treatment A and treatment B; this would be the between-subject information. The assumption that the subject effect is fixed results in treatment information available in subject totals being ignored. To recover the information in subject totals, the subject effects should be considered a random effect. The two estimates of treatment difference are combined based on suitable weights derived from the variance of the two estimators. Suppose that τ_w and τ_b are the estimated treatment difference based on the within-subject and between-subject information respectively. The corresponding variance is σ^2 and σ_s^2 respectively. The combined estimate of treatment difference using weight w is:

$$\tau_c = w\tau_w + (1-w)\tau_b$$

with variance:

$$\sigma_{\tau_c}^2 = w^2\sigma^2 + (1-w)^2\sigma_s^2$$

The variance is minimized if $w = \sigma_s^2/(\sigma^2 + \sigma_s^2)$ which is the intraclass correlation (Senn, 2002). Since the weight itself is estimated, not accounting for this leads to an underestimation of variance for the combined estimator. The analysis described is in practice implemented in a more efficient manner when we use the mixed model approach with subject as a random effect. Here, the estimation is based on a restricted maximum likelihood approach in which the variance components are first estimated, and these are then used to estimate the fixed effects. To address the bias due to the underestimation of the standard error and also to ensure that the correct residual degrees of freedom is used during the testing, the adjustment method proposed by Kenward and Roger (1997) is recommended. The adjustment is mainly impactful for a small sample size but it is a recommended practice to use this as the default method. The recovery of between-subject information is usually not of interest due to the lack of precision. It could be of interest in the case of a less-efficient design like BIB crossover. If the intraclass correlation is relatively small, then it could be worthwhile to incorporate the between-subject information. Otherwise, it might be better to consider the subject effects as fixed. The adjustment proposed by Kenward and Roger is available in the SAS procedure PROC MIXED via the option DDFM = KENWARDROGER redundant.

   A sample size calculation procedure for three-treatment two-period BIB crossover designs is available (Lui and Chang, 2015). The procedure can be used for the case in which we have two active treatments and placebo and the primary concern is to compare the two active treatments against the placebo. The sample size for other BIB crossover designs can be assessed through simulation.

In some situations where BIB design is not available, an alternative design called partially BIB design could be considered. In this design, some pairs of treatments which are more important occur more frequently than others. Details of this design will not be discussed in this chapter. Another type of crossover called n-of-1 design will be discussed in Section 4.3.5.

4.3.5 The *n* of 1 Trial Designs

N of 1 trials are increasingly proposed as alternative designs to RCTs. They are initially proposed to test the treatment effect on individual subjects. Such trials are often multicycle, crossover comparisons of an intervention and a control treatment. Just like crossover trials, n of 1 trials could improve the efficiency and save sample size in rare disease settings as subjects serve as their own controls. Such designs are desirable if there is less within-patient variability in a treatment response than there is between-patient variability. In such cases, outcome estimates will have less variance and the study design will require a less sample size. However, these study designs are applicable only in the situation where there is a relatively rapid response to the intervention, the response disappears relatively soon after the intervention is withdrawn, and the participant's overall condition does not change during the intervention or post-intervention periods. As such, n-of-1 designs are useful to evaluate the treatment of chronic stable conditions, such as attention-deficit/hyperactivity disorder, chronic pain, and arthritis (Nikels, 2017; Huber et al., 2007; Shaffer et al., 2015; Sung et al., 2007; Stunnenberg et al., 2015).

Although n of 1 trials are similar to crossover trials, there are key differences between them. Crossover trials usually use only one treatment cycle between the new intervention and current gold standard care. N of 1 trials typically use multiple cycles which increase the power of the study. N of 1 trials can deliver immediate and clear information about both a patient's response to a treatment and the combined patients' responses (population effect). Zucker et al. (2010) discussed three analytical methods for combining data from n of 1 trials (1) summary data meta-analysis, (2) linear mixed models using maximum likelihood (individual subject data), and (3) BHMs. The summary data meta-analysis approach estimates the pooled treatment effect by combining summary data from each subject using a weighted average.

An n of 1 trial was designed to evaluate the effect of active treatment against placebo in subjects with cystic fibrosis. This is a randomized, double-blinded, placebo-controlled, multiple within-subject crossover study. Subjects were randomized in a 1:1:1:1 ratio to 1 of the 4 treatment sequences as shown in Table 4.9.

Let Y_{ij} be the observed ppFEV1 on the ith subject and jth period. For the summary data meta-analysis approach, the estimate of the pooled treatment effect can be computed as the weighted average $\hat{\mu} = \sum_{i=1}^{n} \frac{w_i y_i}{\sum_{i=1}^{n} w_i}$ of the

TABLE 4.9

Treatment Sequences in N of 1 Design

	Cycle 1	Cycle 1	Cycle 2	Cycle 2
Sequence	Period 1	Period 2	Period 1	Period 2
1	Treatment	Placebo	Treatment	Placebo
2	Treatment	Placebo	Placebo	Treatment
3	Placebo	Treatment	Treatment	Placebo
4	Placebo	Treatment	Placebo	Treatment

individual estimates y_i with weight w_i where y_i is the treatment effect estimated based on the data from individual subject i. In a fixed-effect model, it is assumed that the true mean effect for each individual subject is the same and the weights are set to be $w_i = \dfrac{1}{\sigma_i^2}$ where σ_i^2 is the measurement error for subject i, which can be estimated based on the data from individual subject i. In a random-effect model, each individual subject is assumed to have a different effect μ_i that follow a common distribution $N(\mu, \tau_b^2)$. Therefore, the weights are set to be $w_i = \dfrac{1}{\tau_b^2 + \sigma_i^2}$ in which σ_i^2 represents within-subject measurement error and τ_b^2 captures the between-subject variability.

The second approach is to combine individual subject data using a linear mixed model. Let Y_i denote the vector of the responses for individual subject i. The general model is often described as:

$$Y_i = X_i \, \theta_i + \bigcup$$

where ϵ_i has a normal distribution $N(0, \Sigma)$ and θ_i follows normal $N(0, D)$.

In the cystic fibrosis example, there is only one active treatment and two treatment cycles. A simple random slope model for the cystic fibrosis trial, where the only covariate is treatment, is as follows:

$$Y_{ij} = \alpha_i + \beta_i X_{ij} + e_{ij}$$

where e_{ij} has a normal distribution $N(0, \sigma_i^2)$, α_i follows a normal distribution $N(\alpha, \tau_\alpha^2)$ and β_i normal $N(\beta, \tau_\beta^2)$, $X_{ij} = 0$ for placebo and $X_{ij} = 1$ for active treatment. For this model, the random error e_{ij} is assumed to be independent of each other. The correlation between the observations from the same subject is expressed by the random effects α_i and β_i.

The other approach to analyze n of 1 trials is BHMs. Bayesian methods provide a formal way to incorporate the prior information into the current trial. The other advantage of the Bayesian approach is that it enables a probability statement about the treatment effect estimate under non-informative prior. For the cystic fibrosis trial, the primary endpoint is the absolute change from baseline in percent-predicted FEV1 (ppFEV1). The treatment effect is represented by the absolute change from cycle baseline in ppFEV1 for active treatment minus absolute change from cycle baseline in ppFEV1 for placebo. Let $\tilde{y}_{ij}$ be the response (difference between active treatment and placebo) for the ith subject in cycle j, $i = 1,\ldots,n, j = 1,2,$ where n is the total number of subjects. Assume $\tilde{y}_{ij}$ follow a normal distribution with mean μ_i and variance $\tilde{\sigma}_i^2$. The individual estimate of the effect from each subject is given by the sample mean $\bar{y}_i$ which follows a normal distribution $N\left(\mu_i, \dfrac{\tilde{\sigma}_i^2}{2}\right)$. The subject mean μ_i is assumed to be normal $N(\mu, \tau^2)$ where μ denotes the population mean treatment effect and is assumed to have a non-informative uniform flat prior distribution, the between-subject variance τ^2 is assumed to have a non-informative inverse gamma prior distribution, i.e., $\dfrac{1}{\tau^2} \sim Gamma(0.001, 0.001)$. Given the small number of measurements available for each subject, the within-subject variance is assumed to be proportional to the sample variance, i.e., $\tilde{\sigma}_i^2 = s_i^2\sigma^2$, where s_i^2 represents the sample variance of the subject i and σ^2 is a common constant that has an inverse gamma prior distribution, i.e., $\sigma^2 \sim IG(0.5, 0.5)$. For subjects having missing measurements, the sample variance will be imputed as the average of the sample variance s of the other subjects.

The posterior distribution of the population and individual treatment effects can be obtained using the Monte Carlo Markov Chain sampling. The mean of the population posterior distribution can be interpreted as the population treatment effect. The posterior distribution for each individual subject can also be obtained by combining subject level and population average data. The mean of the individual posterior distributions can be interpreted as the treatment effect for each subject.

N of 1 trials allow the estimate of individual effect and the average treatment effect as well. Multiple repeated assessments on each subject permit the estimation of patient-specific effects and their precision and enable the balance between individual effectiveness and population effectiveness objectives. As in crossover trials, an increase in the treatment periods would improve the study power. However, the gain of having more periods is limited if the within-patient variance is large compared with between-patient variances. Two major limitations of n of 1 design are noted: (1) it is uncertain what proportion of patients will benefit from treatment and (2) insufficient data on adverse effects of treatment are generated. Although increasing the number of periods would improve the precision, patient selection bias might impact the interpretation of the results. As such, if the number of subjects is small, generalization of the population effect estimates from N of 1 trials might be problematic.

Blackston et al. (2019) performed simulation studies to compare n of 1 trials with parallel and crossover RCTs. They showed that the sample sizes required to achieve a target power were lower for n of 1 trials than for parallel and crossover designs. Carryover effects can inflate type I error rate for n of 1 trials similarly to crossover trials. When the samples are not fully representative of the target population, all three designs make an incorrect decision but n of 1 designs make incorrect conclusions far more often due to the increased number of assessments on each subject. One advantage with n of 1 designs is that such designs can identify patients who are outliers for the population of interest.

4.3.6 Population Enrichment Design

The 2019b FDA guidance on enrichment strategies for clinical trials to support the approval of human drugs and biological products provided a comprehensive discussion on the statistical and practical considerations of population enrichment designs (US FDA, 2019). According to the guidance, enrichment is "the prospective use of any patient characteristic to select a study population in which detection of a drug effect (if one is in fact present) is more likely than it would be in an unselected population." Trials can be enriched on baseline characteristics, clinical presentations, biomarkers, or genotypes. Three broad types of clinical trial enrichment strategies defined in the guidance are summarized as follows:

Strategy		Objective
Decrease variability	Choose patients with baseline measurements of a disease or biomarker characterizing the disease in a narrow range and exclude patients whose disease or symptoms improve spontaneously or whose measurements are highly variable	Reduce variability
Prognostic enrichment	Choose patients with a greater likelihood of having a disease-related endpoint event or a substantial worsening in condition	Increase the absolute effect between groups but not the relative effect
Predictive enrichment	Choose patients who are more likely to respond to the drug treatment than other patients with the condition being treated	Increase both the absolute and relative effect size

Complexities in rare diseases include high heterogeneity at the patient level, which leads to a variable progression of the disease and large variability in clinical outcome measures. These challenges are not unique to rare diseases. However, the impacts are aggravated as the commonly used approaches to handle such complexities, such as enrolling a large number of subjects, will no longer be applicable due to the limited number of patients available. Population enrichment designs are particularly attractive for rare diseases as they intend to improve a study's ability to detect a drug's effectiveness, hence supporting smaller sample sizes. When it comes to the use of population enrichment designs, many issues demand critical considerations at the design stage, including the implication of the labeling, generalizability of the trial results to clinical practice, choice of enrichment factor, and existing information available to appropriately define the enrichment factor. For complicated designs, complex statistical methodologies may need to be employed to control the overall false-positive rate and extensive simulations need to be conducted to understand the performance of the study design under different scenarios.

In this section, we focus on the population enrichment designs of confirmatory trials. We discuss the advantages and limitations of various types of enrichment designs, highlight the key design considerations, and illustrate their application in rare disease settings using case studies.

4.3.6.1 Enrichment Design to Decrease Variability

Almost all clinical trials are enrichment designs to decrease non-drug-related heterogeneity. Strategies include but are not limited to the following (1) enrolling a subset of patients who are of more homogeneous characteristics, (2) enrolling patients who are likely to have good compliance with treatment, (3) excluding patients who are unlikely to tolerate the treatment, and (4) utilizing a placebo run-in period to decrease placebo response and spontaneous improvement. While these strategies may reduce the generalizability of the study results to clinical practice, they can decrease the variability, hence allowing for a better chance of demonstrating a treatment effect.

4.3.6.2 Prognostic Enrichment Design

Prognostic enrichment aims to enroll patients with some baseline features that are associated with a higher likelihood of experiencing a poor clinical outcome measure. It is typically used in studies that aim to show a slowed disease progression or a reduced unfavorable outcome. Studies with prognostic enrichment start with enrolling patients with and without the enrichment factor and plan to analyze the subpopulation of patients with the enrichment factor as the primary analysis or one of the primary analyses. The study design focuses on demonstrating a treatment effect in the subpopulation of patients with the enrichment factor. It also allows for the possibility to demonstrate a treatment effect in the overall population via a co-primary endpoint or a secondary endpoint. Randomization is usually stratified by the enrichment factor.

Prognostic enrichment designs have been used in many therapeutic areas such as cardiovascular, oncology, pulmonary, and neurology studies. The key statistical consideration for such trials in the confirmatory trial setting is designing a strategy to maximize the power while adjusting for multiplicity that arises from testing treatment effects in multiple populations (i.e., overall population and the enriched subpopulation). The proper choice of a strategy depends on the confidence of the treatment effect in the enriched population and the prioritization of the hypotheses corresponding to the populations. Freidlin et al. (2013) and Freidlin and Korn (2014) discussed methodologies for adjusting for multiplicity in such a case. Hu and Dignam (2019) also provided some useful illustrative strategies. Here, we provide a case study of prognostic enrichment design in the rare disease setting.

4.3.6.2.1 Case Study of Prognostic Enrichment Design: The INBUILD Trial in Fibrosing Interstitial Lung Disease with a Progressive Phenotype

Fibrosing interstitial lung disease with a progressive phenotype is a rare type of interstitial lung disease (ILD) (Valeyre et al., 2014). Nintedanib, a multitargeted tyrosine kinase inhibitor that inhibits key pathways involved in lung fibrosis in ILDs, was approved by the FDA in 2020 as the first treatment for this indication. The approval was based on a single phase 3 study named INBUILD featuring prognostic enrichment (Flaherty et al., 2019).

In the INBUILD trial, patients were randomized in a 1:1 ratio to receive either nintedanib or placebo for at least 52 weeks. The primary endpoint was the annual rate of decline in forced vital capacity over 52 weeks, which was an established measure of lung function. An enrichment factor of fibroid pattern was used based on a high-resolution computed tomography (HRCT). The study was enriched with approximately two-thirds of the patients with usual interstitial pneumonia (UIP)-like HRCT pattern and the rest one-third of the patients with other HRCT fibrotic patterns. It was expected that patients with a UIP-like HRCT pattern will have a greater annual rate of decline as compared to patients with other HRCT fibrotic patterns and therefore a larger absolute difference from placebo. The enrichment was used to increase the likelihood of success and was also to overcome the challenge of recruiting many patients with this rare disease. This study was the first prognostic enrichment study in the ILD file that was enriched based on the clinical behavior of the disease rather than the primary clinical diagnosis.

There were two co-primary populations defined for the analyses: the overall population and a subpopulation of patients with HRCT with UIP-like HRCT fibrotic pattern. A Hochberg procedure was used for multiplicity control. The study was to be considered positive if analyses in both co-primary populations are significant at the two-sided 5% level or if the analyses in the overall or the subpopulation are statistically significant at the two-sided 2.5% level. The subgroup of patients in the other HRCT fibrotic patterns was not expected to have sufficient power to achieve statistical significance at the study design stage.

The study met its primary endpoint in both the overall population and the subpopulation, with the nintedanib showing a slowed loss of pulmonary function as compared to the placebo. The primary endpoint in the other HRCT subpopulation was also nominally significant, albeit having a smaller magnitude of the treatment effect. Nintedanib was approved for the overall population based on these results.

4.3.6.3 Predictive Enrichment Design

Predictive enrichment aims to select a subgroup of patients who are more likely to respond to the treatment based on enrichment factors, allowing for increased efficiency or feasibility and an enhanced benefit–risk relationship. Unlike prognostic enrichment in which patients are chosen to have a greater likelihood of having a disease-related endpoint event or a substantial worsening in condition, predictive enrichment selects patients based on a specific aspect of physiology or a disease characteristic that is associated with the target therapy's mechanism. If the enrichment factor is related to the magnitude of the treatment effect, the predictive enrichment design has the advantage of enhanced power and therefore allows for a smaller sample size. The disadvantages of such a trial design are related to generalizability and potentially lack of information in the excluded subgroup.

When there is good evidence that an enrichment factor will predict treatment response, the study can be enriched directly by enrolling only patients with the enrichment factor. Such enrichment is typically based on genetic or proteomic markers and there are many cases in oncology. Examples in the rare disease setting include the TRIVE and ENVISION trials of ivacaftor for cystic fibrosis patients with the G551D mutation (Ramsey et al., 2011; Davies et al., 2013), and the VALOR trial of Tofersen for patients with ALS associated with SOD1 mutation (a rare genetic form of ALS; Miller et al., 2020).

When there are uncertainties around whether a specific enrichment factor will predict the treatment response, the response to the treatment will need to be evaluated in the study. According to the FDA guidance (FDA, 2019b), there are two general approaches for such cases. One approach is to choose patients who can respond by finding a genetic or physiological characteristic that predicts response to the test treatment via an unblinded interim analysis. Such design is typically referred to as the adaptive enrichment design and it is discussed in Section 4.3.6.4. The other approach is to test the overall population in an open-label treatment period and then withdraw the treatment for responders via the so-called randomized withdrawal design and the design will be further discussed in Section 4.3.7.

4.3.6.4 Adaptive Enrichment Design

The adaptive enrichment design is a type of design that aims to identify patients who would benefit most from the treatment by incorporating the information collected during the trial via an unblinded interim analysis. Adaptive enrichment designs are typically two-stage designs that start with a broad enrollment criterion in the first stage. After the prespecified unblinded interim analysis, the study may be terminated for futility, continue as planned, or continue by enrolling patients only in a subgroup defined by the enrichment factor in the second stage. Such designs are particularly useful when there is some biological basis to support a treatment effect in the subgroup of patients with the enrichment factor. Nonetheless, it remains unclear whether the subgroup of patients without the enrichment factor may also benefit from the treatment. The interim analysis helps verify the predictive capability of the enrichment factor and determine whether the remainder of the study should be restricted to the subgroup in which the treatment was perceived as effective. The final statistical analysis of the data would be based on data from the two stages with strategies to prevent the inflation of the type I error rate.

Key statistical issues are around the control of the type I error rate and the adjustment of the potential estimation bias in treatment effects (Thall, 2021). Simulations are important at the design stage to delineate the operating characteristics of the study design, such as the type I error rate, the power, the expected sample size and trial duration, the extent of bias in treatment effect estimates, and the coverage of confidence intervals. A case study of adaptive enrichment design is discussed below.

4.3.6.4.1 *Case Study of the Adaptive Enrichment Design: The TAPPAS Trial in Angiosarcoma*

Angiosarcoma (AS) is an aggressive and ultrarare cancer that develops in the inner lining of the blood vessels and lymph vessels, with an estimated incidence of 1,000 patients per year in the United States (Mehta et al., 2019). The TAPPAS trial was a two-stage adaptive enrichment phase III trial of TRC105 and pazopanib versus pazopanib alone in patients with advanced AS. It was the first randomized phase III trial in AS and the study design incorporated input from the FDA and EMA. Patients with two AS subtypes (cutaneous and non-cutaneous) were enrolled in the first stage of the trial and randomization was stratified by AS subtype and the number of lines of prior therapy for AS (Mehta et al., 2019).

The study had a planned unblinded interim analysis by an independent DMC to allow for sample size re-estimation or population enrichment of patients with cutaneous AS. Population enrichment was planned as there was some suggestion of greater tumor sensitivity to TRC105 in the cutaneous subgroup. The interim analysis was to determine the conditional power for the full population (CP_F) and the conditional power for the cutaneous subpopulation (CP_S). Based on the interim analysis, the study was to:

- continue as planned with the full population if in the favorable zone ($CP_F > 95\%$) or unfavorable zone ($CP_F < 30\%$),
- continue with the full population and increase sample size and the number of PFS events if in the promising zone ($30\% \leq CP_F \leq 95\%$), and
- continue with the cutaneous subpopulation if in the enrichment zone ($CP_F < 30\%$ and $CP_S \geq 50\%$).

The operating characteristics of the design were evaluated by simulation. The final analysis was planned to be based on combining the p-values from the two stages. To preserve the family-wise type I error rate, statistical adjustment was needed to account for the multiplicity due to the selection of either the full population or cutaneous subpopulation in the interim analysis, as well as for possible changes in the sample size. The method of Jenkins et al. (2010) was chosen and detailed multiplicity adjustment was discussed in the supplemental material of Mehta et al (2019).

The study was discontinued after the interim analysis due to futility. The trial did not meet its primary endpoint and showed no benefit compared to TRC105 and pazopanib versus pazopanib alone in patients with advanced AS (Jones et al., 2019).

4.3.7 Randomized Withdrawal Design

The randomized withdrawal design is a type of predictive enrichment design (FDA, 2019b). In a randomized withdrawal trial, patients receive the test treatment during the open-label period, and responders are then randomly assigned to continue with the test treatment or with the placebo in the randomized withdrawal period. The trial is enriched with people who are responsive to the treatment.

The randomized withdrawal design is very attractive from the enrollment perspective as subjects are expected to receive a placebo for a reduced or minimized period. For some diseases where the symptoms are severe, patients are reluctant to come off the standard treatment, and an add-on design is not feasible, the randomized withdrawal design may be the only option to test the efficacy of the new treatment. For example, the randomized withdrawal design was found to be the only viable design option to assess the efficacy of vixotrigine for the treatment of trigeminal neuralgia, a rare chronic pain condition (Kotecha et al., 2020; Zakrzewska et al., 2017).

The disadvantages are related to the difficulty to generalize the results to clinical practice because the effectiveness of the treatment is only demonstrated in patients who have already shown a response to the treatment. Therefore, the randomized withdrawal design is commonly used to establish the long-term maintenance effect of treatment. Recently, there is increasing use of the design to establish the efficacy of a new treatment either jointly with studies of conventional designs or on its own, especially in the rare disease setting.

Key design considerations of a randomized withdrawal design include appropriate treatment duration for the open-label period, the criteria for responders that will allow the population to show the best treatment effect, and the actions to maintain blinding for patients who switched from treatment to placebo in the randomized withdrawal period.

Two case studies are discussed below to illustrate the application of the design.

4.3.7.1 Randomized Withdrawal Design Case Study 1: The ICE Trial in Chronic Inflammatory Demyelinating Polyneuropathy

Chronic inflammatory demyelinating polyneuropathy (CIDP) is a rare neurological disorder, with an estimated incidence of 1–9 per 1,000, 000 adults in the United States (Langhlin et al., 2009). IGIV-C is an intravenous immunoglobulin approved for the treatment of CIDP. Approval for this indication was based on a pivotal study that included two randomized study periods (the efficacy and randomized withdrawal period) to assess whether IGIV-C was more effective than placebo and whether long-term administration of IGIV-C could maintain long-term benefits (Hughes et al., 2008). In the double-blind efficacy period, patients were randomized to IGIV-C or placebo and received treatment for 24 weeks. Patients who completed the efficacy period and responded to the therapy were eligible for entry into a double-bind randomized withdrawal period to be randomized to IGIV-C or placebo. The primary endpoint was met with significantly more patients being responded to IGIV-C as compared to placebo in the efficacy period. During the randomized withdrawal period, patients re-randomized to IVIG-C experienced a significantly longer time to relapse compared to those receiving placebo.

In this case, IGIV-C was approved based on the results not only from the efficacy period but also from the randomized withdrawal period. IGIV-C is indicated for the treatment of CIDP to improve neuromuscular disability and impairment and for maintenance therapy to prevent relapse (IGIVnex Product Monograph, 2019).

4.3.7.2 Randomized Withdrawal Design Case Study 2: The VALO Trial in Pachyonychia Congenita

Pachyonychia congenita (PC) is a rare, chronically debilitating, and lifelong genetic disease. Patients with PC experience extreme pain and difficulty with ambulation. Over 9,000 individuals are estimated to be living with PC in the United States (Gallagher et al., 2019).

The VALO study was a multicenter, two-stage, randomized withdrawal design to evaluate the efficacy of PTX-022 in adults with moderate-to-severe PC. Patients in this study went through a 4-week run-in period followed by a phase II open-label treatment period in which they received PTX-022 once daily for 12 weeks. At the end of phase II, patients who met a re-defined clinical response criterion were seamlessly enrolled into a randomized withdrawal phase III period of 12 weeks and assigned to one of the three arms: two dose regimens of PTX-022 or placebo. Here, the randomized withdrawal period aims to establish the efficacy as compared to assessing the maintenance effect as in Case Study 1.

In the phase II portion of the study, PTX-022 demonstrated a statistically significant improvement on the primary endpoint, which contrasted the last 2 weeks of the phase II open-label treatment period to the last 2 weeks of the run-in period. However, the primary endpoint was not met in the phase III randomized withdrawal portion of the study. The pooled two-dose regimens of PTX-022 did not show a treatment effect on the primary endpoint compared to placebo (Palvella Therapeutics, 2020).

4.3.8 Totality of Evidence Analysis of Clinical Trials of Rare Diseases

4.3.8.1 Combining Endpoints for Totality-of-Evidence Analyses

It may not be uncommon in rare disease clinical trials to have insufficient power to declare treatment superiority for the endpoint which is of the greatest ultimate interest. Such an endpoint may be difficult to assess in a reasonable time frame when only a limited number of patients are available. Overall survival or time to end-stage kidney disease are examples of endpoints that are very important to patients and clinicians, yet difficult to power in the rare disease setting.

One approach to mitigate the issue and demonstrate the value of novel therapy is a pre-planned "totality-of-evidence" analysis. Apart from any limited amount of data available on the patient's primary outcome, additional clinically meaningful endpoints may be available. These endpoints may not be individually powered either. However, it may be that a constellation of endpoints substantially trending in a favorable direction lends credence to the proposition that the novel therapy has value. We call this a totality-of-evidence analysis. Ristl et al. (2019) gave a comprehensive overview of various methods, which are mostly data-type specific. Note that this analysis may commonly be a supportive analysis conducted after a statistically and clinically meaningful effect has been demonstrated on a shorter-term endpoint more proximal to the therapy's mechanism of action. For example, the primary endpoint may be the modulation of a biomarker believed to be important to the course of the disease. In that case, the primary endpoint would likely not be included as part of the totality-of-evidence analysis.

In the particular setting of rare disease clinical trials, both the expected treatment effect and the number of variables (endpoints) included may be small to moderate, rather than a zero effect for many variables and a large effect for a small number, as one might expect in genomic studies. Also, we expect the variables in question to have some level of correlation in the same direction, though perhaps not strongly so, or otherwise only one of the strongly correlated variables would be selected for inclusion. Additionally, we focus on approaches that can be robustly applied to various kinds of data (e.g., continuous, binary, ordinal, and time-to-event) since we may not have the luxury of only choosing variables of a certain form. Lastly, we only investigate approaches that test a global null hypothesis that there is no treatment effect on any of the endpoints. We consider the one-sided level $\alpha = 0.025$ test for simplicity. The approaches discussed are with a randomized setting in mind, though some may apply to a nonrandomized setting. It is expected in this setting that the multiple-endpoint analysis would be considered a secondary or supportive analysis. The primary analysis endpoint may be a surrogate or biomarker-based endpoint more proximal to the mechanism of action which is easier, faster, and/or less variable to detect the treatment effect upon than it would be for more incontrovertible clinical endpoints. As failure on this surrogate/biomarker endpoint would be unlikely to result in clinical success, a statistical analysis plan may prespecify that the multiple-endpoint test only be conducted if the primary analysis is significant, obviating multiplicity issues. Hence, in the following summary, no multiplicity adjustment is applied.

We organize the rest of the work as follows. We introduce a subset of approaches to the totality of evidence most relevant to our key considerations in Section 4.3.8.2. We set up a series of simulations comparing various investigated approaches and present the results in Section 4.3.8.3. Finally, we end by discussing some potential additional approaches that may warrant future consideration in Section 4.3.8.4.

4.3.8.2 Selected Approaches to Multiple-Endpoint Analyses

Consider a randomized two-arm clinical trial in which the treatment group (Group 1) is in comparison with a control group (Group 2), where there are n_i patients in group $i = 1$, 2 respectively. Here, we set $n_1 = n_2 = n$ for simplicity. We consider a total of m endpoints are of interest and use the index $k = 1, ..., m$ to indicate the kth endpoint.

4.3.8.2.1 O'Brien's OLS and GLS Statistics

To account for directionality and correlations of endpoints, to test the global hypothesis, O'Brien (1984) proposed two parametric procedures, where all endpoints are assumed to be continuous and share the same non-negative standardized effect size λ. Following this, the multivariate hypothesis tests are integrated into a single hypothesis testing problem:

$$H_0 : \lambda = 0 \ vs. \ H_1 : \lambda > 0.$$

The ordinary least square (OLS) procedure is to strategically form an estimator of λ that equally adds over m endpoints, i.e., $\hat{\lambda}_{OLS} = J^T t$, where J is a $m \times 1$ column vector of all 1s and $t = (t_1, ..., t_m)^T$ being the univariate t-statistics. Thus, the OLS statistic can be written as:

$$t_{OLS} = \frac{\hat{\lambda}_{OLS}}{SE\left(\hat{\lambda}_{OLS}\right)} = \frac{J^T t}{\sqrt{J^T \hat{R} J}},$$

where $\hat{R}$ is the sample correlation of the standardized t-statistics.

Alternatively, unlike λ_{OLS} that assigns the weight equally, the GLS estimate is formed by adding the weights equivalent to the row sums, resulting in a possibly more powerful test statistic:

$$t_{GLS} = \frac{\hat{\lambda}_{GLS}}{SE\left(\hat{\lambda}_{GLS}\right)} = \frac{J^T \hat{R}^{-1} t}{\sqrt{J^T \hat{R}^{-1} J}}.$$

One can approximate intractable OLS and GLS statistics via the t-distribution with certain degrees of freedom (df), denoted by v. Various estimates of v have been proposed in the literature. Logan and Tamhane (2004) proposed $v = 0.5(n_1 + n_2 - 2)(1 + 1/m^2)$, which we adopt throughout as it is generally conservative in most simulation scenarios (Dallow et al., 2008). Moreover, because of the likely appearance of negative weights due to an irregular correlation structure in t_{GLS} according to Pocock et al. (1987) and its possible failure to preserve the type I error rate, Dallow et al. (2008), we only consider the OLS-type procedure.

4.3.8.2.2 Extensions to the OLS

Since our interest is a mixture of data types, modifications of the original O'Brien's test, which only considers continuous endpoints, are needed. Sun et al. (2012) proposed the average of the z-score approach. It first converts different data types to the corresponding pseudo-continuous measures, i.e., the z-scores. For continuous, binary, and ordinal types, the z-scores are obtained by subtracting the pooled groups' mean and dividing the pooled groups' standard deviation. For time-to-event endpoints, the censoring status and survival outcomes are altogether transformed into a log-rank score. Then, a Wilcoxon rank-sum test is conducted on the average of aligned z-scores in the same direction. Alternatively, instead of taking the average of aligned z-scores, one can treat them as if they were observed continuous measures and invoke the OLS procedure. By using this approach, we consider the correlation among endpoints more explicitly. Note that both approaches combine the outcome data at the patient level, meaning that the statistic of interest contains explicit individual-level data.

The third extension to O'Brien's OLS procedure is to combine test statistics at the endpoint level while considering correlations among test statistics. More specifically, one can first test each endpoint univariately with any test of the researcher's choice, depending on the data types (e.g., t-test, Fisher's exact test, negative binomial model, and log-rank test). The corresponding outputs, i.e., the univariate statistics $t = (t_1,...,t_m)^T$, are combined to form the final statistic of interest in an OLS manner, that is, the sum of individual statistic $J^T t$. For non-t-scale or non-z-scale test statistics, we set $t_k = \phi^{-1}(1 - p_k)$, where ϕ^{-1} is the inverse cumulative distribution function (CDF) of normal distribution and p_k is the p-value from the kth endpoint. As an endpoint-level statistic, we estimate the correlation matrix among individual statistics $\hat{R}$ by permutations. Here, the endpoint-level statistic refers to the final statistic made by (functions of) the univariate test statistics.

4.3.8.2.3 *p-value Combination Approaches*

Another cluster of methods is to combine p-values from a set of m hypotheses. In general, a function of the p-values $H(p_k)$ and a weight w_k are realized, resulting in a statistic of the form $T = \sum w_k H(p_k)$ and then a single p-value is calculated based on the distribution of T for decision-making. The existing approaches include Fisher's p-value combination method by Fisher (1925), where the function $H = -2\ln(p_k)$ with equal weights $w_k = 1$. Stouffer et al. (1949) transformed each p-value p_k back to the equally weighted (i.e., $w_k = 1$) z-scores by setting H as the inverse CDF of normal distribution $\phi^{-1}(p_k)$. Lancaster (1961) constructed $H = \chi^2_{(w_k)}{}^{-1}(1 - p_k)$, that is an inverse CDF of the chi-square distribution with df of w_k. These methods initially assume that the m hypotheses are independent, and each p-value is uniformly distributed on the interval $[0, 1]$ under the null. However, such assumptions are likely not valid for our considered endpoints, and extensions to the dependent case are needed.

Dai et al. (2014) modified the Lancaster (1961) procedure to a dependent case, where the statistic is $T_D = \sum_{k=1}^{m} \chi^2_{(w_k)}{}^{-1}(1 - p_k)$ and the distribution of T_D does not have an explicit analytical form. Throughout the following, we adopt their recommended Satterthwaite method for approximation. Moreover, permutation can be implemented to estimate the correlations among p-values. Without any available information on the weights, we use $w_k = 2$ for all $k = 1,\ldots,m$ per the default from Dai et al. (2014).

Furthermore, Zaykin et al. (2002) modified Fisher's method by truncating the product of p-values below a threshold τ with a focus on smaller p-values, where the statistic for this procedure can be written as $T_Z = \prod_{k=1}^{m} p_k^{I(p_k \leq \tau)}$. Zaykin further extended the procedure to a dependent case and provided a way to calculate the probability of T_Z by employing the Cholesky decomposition and the feature of (approximately) invariant correlation under monotone transformation, given that the correlation structure of p-values is known. When the correlation structure is unknown, similar to T_D, one can estimate them by permutations. While Zaykin et al. (2002) primarily discussed $\tau = 0.05$ in a context of genome analyses with very large m and numerous significant results, here, we set the threshold τ to be 0.5 to only keep the endpoints in the "correct" direction as consistency of effect across endpoints is desirable. Also, note that both the correlated Lancaster's approach by Dai et al. (2014) and the truncated product method by Zaykin et al. (2002) combine test statistics at endpoint level.

4.3.8.2.4 *Generalized Pairwise Comparisons*

The methods we have introduced so far typically handle each endpoint as equally important, which might not be the case where, for example, the endpoints are a mixture of fatal and nonfatal ones. Weighted versions of these methods are available, but the choice of weights may struggle to highlight the relative importance of the endpoints in a way that is easily interpretable and agreeable to regulators and the clinical community in general. To naturally capture the hierarchical feature of endpoints, several methods are proposed, e.g., the Finkelstein–Schoenfeld score (Finkelstein and Schoenfeld, 1999), the win ratio (Pocock et al., 2012), and our focus, the generalized pairwise comparisons (GPC) by Buyse (2010).

In the GPC approach which is an extension of the U-statistic for the Wilcoxon-Mann-Whitney test, a hierarchy of m prioritized endpoints in mixed data types is first established, with endpoint 1 being the highest priority level and m being the lowest priority level. Within each kth endpoint, a clinically justifiable rule is further installed to compare the outcome from a pair of individuals, denoted as $a = 1, \ldots, n_1$ and $b = 1, \ldots, n_2$ from group 1 and group 2, respectively. Specifically, we denote two indicators on kth endpoint outcome between the current individual pair (a, b):

$$u_{ab}(k) = \begin{cases} 1, & \text{If the } k\text{th outcome is uninformative} \\ 0, & \text{otherwise} \end{cases},$$

$$p_{ab}(k) = \begin{cases} 1, & \text{If the } k^{th} \text{ outcome is favorable (win)} \\ -1, & \text{If the } k^{th} \text{ outcome is unfavorable (loss)} \\ 0, & \text{If the } k^{th} \text{ outcome is neutral (tie)} \end{cases} \text{nd } u_{ab}(h) = 1, \forall h < k$$

Finally, to summarize the total of $n_1 n_2$ pairwise results, the net benefit is defined as:

$$\Delta = \sum_{k \leq m} \delta(k) = \sum_{k \leq m} \frac{\sum_{a=1}^{n_1} \sum_{b=1}^{n_2} p_{ab}(k)}{n_1 n_2} \in (-1, 1),$$

where $\delta(k)$ is a signed proportion representing the fraction of examined $n_1 n_2$ pairs that the treatment is better than the controlled group with respect to the kth endpoint. With being the realization of the totality of evidence across all endpoints, our hypothesis of interest becomes $H_0 : \Delta = 0$. The inference of can be made by the asymptotic theory of U-statistics, permutation, or bootstrap. Here, combines the outcome data at the patient level.

4.3.8.3 Simulations

4.3.8.3.1 Setup

We conducted simulations to compare the operating characteristics of the approaches mentioned in Section 4.3.8.2. The approaches considered are summarized in Table 4.10. For the first objective, we compared the performance of selected methods in simulations where all endpoints of various types were equally powered in favor of the treatment group. We excluded the GPC method for comparison in objective one as it was not as powerful as other methods in our considered simulation scenarios. Additionally, as the second objective, we envisioned a scenario where two endpoints are to be explicitly ordered clinically and possibly unequal effect sizes for each ordered endpoint in assessing the statistical properties of the considered approaches, including the GPC method. In particular, we investigate simulation scenarios under the alternative where the less clinically prioritized endpoint has no or even a negative drug effect.

As we consider a mixture of possibly correlated data types, the data generation is not trivial. Therefore, we adopted the data generation algorithm described in Sun et al. (2012) and Brown and Ezekowitz (2017) to generate the data in an iterative process. Moreover, in objective one, we considered five endpoints: continuous, binary, two ordinals, and time-to-event. For example, the two ordinal endpoints can represent the number of severe pulmonary exacerbations (PEx) and the number of moderate-to-severe PEx, respectively. Also, we anticipated severe events to be clinically more prioritized than moderate-to-severe.

If the drug is efficacious, it is possible to see a decreasing number of severe PEx, "downgrading" and shifting more to moderate-to-severe PEx in the drug group, ultimately leading to a zero or negative effect on the secondly prioritized endpoint. Therefore, we also generated those two ordinal endpoints in the simulations for objective two. In these simulations, we considered the following sample sizes per group to be 20, 30, 50, 100, and 200. We assumed the correlations to be the same among all endpoints and set them to 0, 0.3, and 0.5 to illustrate no, moderate, and strong correlations. For

TABLE 4.10

Summary of Considered Approaches

Method	Summary
z-score nonP	The nonparametric average of the z-scores approach by Sun et al. (2012). Convert the actual data to "pseudo-continuous" z-scores. Nonparametric test on the average of z-scores. Combine outcome data at the patient level.
z-score OLS	Convert the actual data to "pseudo-continuous" z-scores. Parametric OLS on individual z-score. Combine outcome data at the patient level.
Hybrid OLS	Test on a univariate endpoint. Parametric OLS on the individual statistic. Combine test statistics at the endpoint level.
Correlated Lancaster	The correlated Lancaster procedure proposed by Dai et al. (2014). Combine *p*-values from univariate tests. Combine test statistics at the endpoint level.
TPM	The truncated product method (TPM) proposed by Zaykin et al. (2002). Combine *p*-values from univariate tests. Truncation of *p*-values below a prespecified threshold. Combine test statistics at the endpoint level.
GPC	The generalized pairwise comparisons (GPC) by Buyse (2010). Extension to the *U*-statistics. Pairwise comparison on prioritized endpoints. Difference between proportions of #wins and #losses. Combine outcome data at the patient level.

the time-to-event outcome, we fixed the censoring month to 24 for simplicity, resulting in about 70% censoring for the study to represent the common situation in which an endpoint of strong clinical importance is not completely mature in the time frame of the current study analyses.

We assessed the operating characteristics of the (empirical) type I error rate and power in the hypothesis testing framework. The type I error rate was evaluated with no effect for all considered endpoints. As for the power, we set the effect size of each endpoint to achieve 30% power at a sample size per arm of 100 and 200. We generated 10,000 datasets with 500 permutations per dataset for correlation estimation purposes among approaches that combine test statistics at the endpoint level for each scenario.

4.3.8.3.2 Results

We present the simulation results in Tables 4.11 and 4.12 and Figure 4.2 and discuss some important implications in the succeeding paragraphs.

TABLE 4.11

Comparison of Type I Error for the Nonparametric Average of z-scores ("z-score nonP"), the OLS Version of z-scores ("z-score OLS"), the Sum of the Individual Test Statistic ("Hybrid OLS"), Dai's Approach ("Correlated Lancaster", $w_k = 2$), and Zakin's Truncated Product Method ("TPM", $\tau = 0.5$)

		Sample Size Per Arm				
Method	Correlation	20	30	50	100	200
z-score nonP	0	0.0231	0.0228	0.0257	0.0225	0.0246
z-score OLS		0.0226	0.0215	0.0253	0.0231	0.0248
Hybrid OLS (Bin = Fisher)		0.0171	0.0175	0.0211	0.0198	0.0224
Hybrid OLS (Bin = z-score)		0.0229	0.0225	0.0257	0.0234	0.0249
Correlated Lancaster		0.0227	0.0209	0.0227	0.0245	0.0246
TPM		0.0201	0.0208	0.0219	0.0233	0.0239
z-score nonP	0.3	0.0260	0.0254	0.0275	0.0245	0.0244
z-score OLS		0.0262	0.0258	0.0270	0.0253	0.0252
Hybrid OLS (Bin = Fisher)		0.0209	0.0214	0.0241	0.0233	0.0230
Hybrid OLS (Bin = z-score)		0.0268	0.0255	0.0277	0.0253	0.0249
Correlated Lancaster		0.0250	0.0237	0.0268	0.0253	0.0263
TPM		0.0280	0.0242	0.0277	0.0275	0.0274
z-score nonP	0.5	0.0267	0.0254	0.0272	0.0218	0.0267
z-score OLS		0.0268	0.0259	0.0272	0.0237	0.0258
Hybrid OLS (Bin = Fisher)		0.0217	0.0237	0.0238	0.0214	0.0244
Hybrid OLS (Bin = z-score)		0.0271	0.0268	0.0275	0.0242	0.0262
Correlated Lancaster		0.0269	0.0266	0.0271	0.0243	0.0249
TPM		0.0228	0.0268	0.0263	0.0247	0.0259

Two variations of the "Hybrid OLS" where the binary endpoint is tested by Fisher's exact test or treated as a continuous measure of z-scores are used. Five endpoints are considered: continuous, binary, two ordinals, and time-to-event.

TABLE 4.12

Comparison of Power (Probability of Rejecting the Global Null) for the Nonparametric Average of z-scores ("z-score nonP"), the OLS Version of z-scores ("z-score OLS"), the Sum of the Individual Test Statistic ("Hybrid OLS"), Dai's Approach ("Correlated Lancaster", $w_k = 2$), and Zaykins Truncated Product Method ("TPM", $\tau = 0.5$)

Method	Correlation	Sample Size per Arm (Univariate 30% Power at Sample Size Per Arm = 200)					Sample Size Per Arm (Univariate 30% Power at Sample Size Per Arm = 100)				
		20	30	50	100	200	20	30	50	100	200
z-score nonP	0	0.2052	0.2888	0.4576	0.7483	0.9594	0.3554	0.5127	0.7420	0.9601	0.9996
z-score OLS		0.2072	0.2985	0.4748	0.7749	0.9696	0.3696	0.5355	0.7693	0.9697	0.9999
Hybrid OLS (Bin = Fisher)		0.1679	0.2598	0.4394	0.7571	0.9657	0.3165	0.4902	0.7443	0.9649	0.9998
Hybrid OLS (Bin = z-score)		0.2089	0.3051	0.4796	0.7764	0.9690	0.3777	0.5411	0.7754	0.9700	0.9999
Correlated Lancaster		0.1771	0.2637	0.4264	0.7215	0.9542	0.3224	0.4796	0.7247	0.9534	0.9997
TPM		0.1672	0.2496	0.4192	0.7192	0.9550	0.3037	0.4649	0.7160	0.9545	0.9996
z-score nonP	0.3	0.1174	0.1567	0.2378	0.4314	0.7178	0.1992	0.2824	0.4320	0.7179	0.9546
z-score OLS		0.1216	0.1623	0.2482	0.4516	0.7498	0.2034	0.2926	0.4500	0.7442	0.9655
Hybrid OLS (Bin = Fisher)		0.1017	0.1440	0.2313	0.4354	0.7419	0.1743	0.2691	0.4277	0.7337	0.9628
Hybrid OLS (Bin = z-score)		0.1216	0.1640	0.2512	0.4524	0.7520	0.2057	0.2962	0.4537	0.7460	0.9656
Correlated Lancaster		0.1214	0.1628	0.2484	0.4461	0.7495	0.1980	0.2902	0.4476	0.7490	0.9649
TPM		0.1148	0.1543	0.2353	0.4248	0.7272	0.1864	0.2698	0.4205	0.7190	0.9552
z-score nonP	0.5	0.0953	0.1284	0.1841	0.3308	0.5800	0.1552	0.2119	0.3310	0.5956	0.8679
z-score OLS		0.0994	0.1344	0.1959	0.3454	0.6059	0.1627	0.2212	0.3426	0.6070	0.8864
Hybrid OLS (Bin = Fisher)		0.0876	0.1229	0.1824	0.3319	0.5986	0.1420	0.2015	0.3280	0.5966	0.8830
Hybrid OLS (Bin = z-score)		0.1013	0.1358	0.1989	0.3472	0.6079	0.1641	0.2250	0.3469	0.6104	0.8877
Correlated Lancaster		0.1002	0.1397	0.1985	0.3478	0.6179	0.1638	0.2249	0.3508	0.6125	0.8960
TPM		0.0943	0.1242	0.1741	0.3106	0.5741	0.1449	0.1968	0.3130	0.5582	0.8641

Two variations of the "Hybrid OLS" where the binary variable is tested by Fisher's exact test or treated as a continuous measure of z-scores are used. Five endpoints are considered: continuous, binary, two ordinals, and time-to-event.

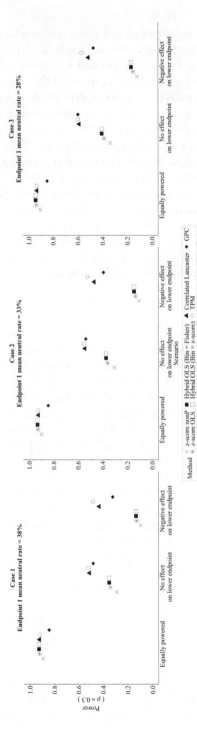

FIGURE 4.2

Comparison of power (probability of rejecting the global null) for the nonparametric average of z-scores ("z-score nonP"), the OLS version of z-scores ("z-score OLS"), the sum of the individual test statistic ("Hybrid OLS"), Dai's approach ("correlated Lancaster", $w_k = 0.5$), correlated Lancaster" ("correlated Lancaster", $w_k = 2$), and Zaykins TPM ("TPM", $\tau = 0.5$). Different simulation cases represent various neutral (uninformative) rates at the higher prioritized endpoint. Two clinically prioritized endpoints are considered (1) the ordinal endpoint that can represent the number of severe PEx and (2) the ordinal endpoint that can represent the number of moderate-to-severe PEx. The sample size per arm is $n = 50$. The correlation between two endpoints is $\rho = 0.3$.

4.3.8.3.3 Type I Error Rate

From Table 4.11, when there is no correlation among endpoints, the methods control the type I error rate comfortably below the 0.025 level. As the correlation increases, methods such as the correlated Lancaster and truncated product method (TPM) method generally become slightly liberal, especially at smaller sample sizes. This is possibly due to incorporating p-values of non-continuous endpoints and the approximation procedures using smaller sample sizes. We set the number of permutations at 500 because it is mainly used for estimating parameters (i.e., correlation matrix) rather than eliciting the empirical distribution of the test statistics. However, increasing the number of permutations (we also considered permutations of 1,000 and 2,000) does not change the results notably (results not shown). We also display two variations of the Hybrid OLS, where the binary endpoint is analyzed by Fisher's exact method ("Bin = Fisher") or treated as continuous z-scores after standardization ("Bin = z-score"). The results show that the former is comparably more conservative at smaller sample sizes. We observe a similar trend in variations of the correlated Lancaster and TPM method.

4.3.8.3.4 Power

For objective one, the results are similar between the two scenarios with different effect sizes, as displayed in Table 4.12. The z-score OLS is universally better powered than its nonparametric counterpart z-score nonP. Also, with the elimination of the conservativeness, the z-score version of the Hybrid OLS is more powerful than its Fisher's exact test version. Generally, at a smaller sample size and when there is no correlation, the z-score-based methods (z-score nonP and z-score OLS) along with the Hybrid OLS (z-score version) outperform the p-value combination approaches. On the other hand, the correlated Lancaster procedure becomes marginally more powerful than the rest at a higher correlation. Under the considered scenarios where all endpoints are equally powered in the same direction, it is unlikely that we observe a large portion of tests to be in the "wrong" direction, i.e., $p_k \geq \tau = 0.5$ under the alternative. Therefore, the TPM is expected to be the least powerful method in considered scenarios. However, due to its truncation feature, the TPM will gain more power under the scenarios when including endpoints with no/negative drug effects, as seen in Figure 4.2. Lastly, it is interesting that the global test's power decreases with the increase of correlation, regardless of methods, which aligns with findings from previous investigations by Deltuvaite-Thomas and Burzykowski (2021) and Senn and Bretz (2007). Overall, many of the procedures perform similarly, and the choice of approach for any particular study may not be driven by the type I error rate or power considerations.

We display the results for the second objective in Figure 4.2. When the two investigated ordinal endpoints with explicit clinical orders are equally powered, the GPC method has the least power. However, in situations where the less prioritized endpoint has no or negative drug effect, the considered methods divide into two clusters: the OLS-type and non-OLS-type (including the GPC), and the latter of which is clearly more powerful. Furthermore, the power difference gap between the two clusters of approaches becomes larger when the less prioritized endpoint is more in the "wrong" direction. As expected, we observe more power gain for the GPC when fewer ties are present in the higher-level endpoint.

On the other hand, the TPM procedure is comparably robust to the neutral (tie) rate and consistently more powerful than the rest of the non-OLS-type approaches. This is because the TPM tends to "remove" endpoints that are not in favor of treatment while other approaches still include them in the final statistic, leading to a decrease in power. Moreover, one can anticipate that when the clinical orders of endpoints are debatable, the TPM method is likely to preserve the power while the GPC could lose power considerably. In conclusion, when the combined endpoints are of different effect sizes or possibly in opposite directions, the non-OLS-type approaches, especially the TPM procedure, can be considered.

4.3.8.4 Discussion

To conduct the totality-of-evidence analysis in testing the global null that the investigational drug has no effect on any of the multiple endpoints, we have introduced a series of methods that either combine the outcome data at the patient level or combine the test statistics at the endpoint level, the latter of which needs further permutations for correlation estimation in practice.

Further integration of methods can be considered. For example, one can incorporate the GPC to capture more information about PEx into the Hybrid OLS, correlated Lancaster, or TPM procedure. The simulation study shows that different methods maintain distinct characteristics under various scenarios. Therefore, before settling on a particular method, researchers must thoroughly assess the situation that they are in. For example, what are the anticipated correlations among endpoints? Is there a clinically justifiable order of importance among endpoints? What do the profile of individual effect sizes look like?

Moreover, the feasibility of implementing a totality-of-evidence analysis warrants careful evaluation, and aggregation of information may not always be a good idea. Consider two standard normal continuous endpoints as an illustrative example. When one endpoint's effect size is much smaller than the other, combining such might result in power loss compared to a single univariate test. In fact, under certain special cases, Dallow et al. (2008) presented an analytical inequality demonstrating circumstances in which adding additional endpoints would increase the power. For example, to allow O'Brien's OLS to outperform the univariate t-test on Endpoint 1 (effect size of 0.396 that corresponds to 50% power), the effect size of the second endpoint needs to be at least $\left[\sqrt{2*(1+\rho)}-1\right]*0.396$, corresponding to 41.4%,

61.2%, and 73.2% of Endpoint 1's effect size for $\rho = 0$, 0.3, and 0.5, respectively. It may be worth noting that, in circumstances where this form of the totality-of-evidence analysis adds value, we find the equal effect assumption (such as in O'Brien's approach) generally somewhat reasonable. If any of the endpoints were viewed as having either quite poor or quite strong individual power, that endpoint would likely either not be included in the analysis or the only endpoint selected (conventional analysis conducted). Lastly, for multiple-endpoint analysis, sample size calculation generally requires simulation, especially when the endpoints are of different types. However, in cases where the endpoints are all continuous, we may be able to carry out the standard sample size calculation for O'Brien's OLS and GLS as long as the t-distribution (Dallow et al., 2008) or z-distribution (Dmitrienko et al., 2009) can approximate the corresponding statistics well enough.

Given all considerations and discussion above, we believe it is important to have several practical options available for analyzing clinical trials with multiple endpoints.

References

Agresti, A. (2013). *Categorical Data Analysis*. 3rd Edition, John Wiley & Sons Inc., Hoboken.

Alemayehu, D, Levenstein, M, Knirsch, C. (2014). Statistical considerations for clinical trials in rare diseases. *The Journal of Rare Disorders*, 2(1), 18–22.

Andersen, P. K., Borgan, O, Gill, R. D., & Keiding, N. (1991). *Statistical Models Based on Counting Processes*. Springer, New York.

Baghfalaki, T., & Ganjali, M. (2020). A transition model for analyzing multivariate longitudinal data using Gaussian copula approach. *AStA Advances in Statistical Analysis*, 104, 169–223.

Barker, A. D., Sigman, C. C., Kelloff, G. J., Hylton, N. M., Berry, D. A., & Esserman, L. (2009). I-SPY 2: An adaptive breast cancer trial design in the setting of neoadjuvant chemotherapy. *Clinical Pharmacology & Therapeutics*, 86(1), 97–100.

Barnes, P. J., Pocock, S. J., Magnussen, H., Iqbal, A., Kramer, B., Higgins, M., & Lawrence, D. (2010). Integrating indacaterol dose selection in a clinical study in COPD using an adaptive seamless design. *Pulmonary Pharmacology & Therapeutics*, 23(3), 165–171.

Bauer, P., & Kieser, M. (1999). Combining different phases in the development of medical treatments within a single trial. *Statistics in Medicine, 18*, 1833–1848.

Bauer, P., Koenig, F., Brannath, W., & Posch, M. (2010). Selection and bias - two hostile brothers. *Statistics in Medicine, 29*(1), 1–13.

Bazzano, A. T., Mangione-Smith, R., Schonlau, M., Suttorp, M.J., & Brook, R.H. (2009). Off-label prescribing to children in the United States outpatient setting. *Academic pediatrics*, 9(2): 81–88. doi: 10.1016/j.acap.2008.11.010. Epub 2009 Feb 11. PMID: 19329098.

Berry, M. S., Broglio, K. R., Groshen, S., & Berry D. B. (2013). Bayesian hierarchical modeling of patient subpopulations: Efficient designs of Phase II oncology clinical trials. *Clinical Trials*, 10(5): 720–734.

Berry, S. M., Carlin, B. P., Lee, J. J., & Muller, P. (2010). *Bayesian Adaptive Methods for Clinical Trials*. CRC Press, Boca Raton.

Blackston, J. W., Chapple, A. G., McGree, J. M., McDonald, S., & Nikles, J. (2019). Comparison of aggregated N-of-1 trials with parallel and crossover randomized controlled trials using simulation studies. *Healthcare (Basel)*, 7(4): 137.

Bowden, J., & Glimm, E. (2014). Conditionally unbiased and near unbiased estimation of the selected treatment mean for multi-stage drop-the-losers trials. *Biometrical Journal*, 56, 332–349.

Brown, H., & Prescott, R. (2006). *Applied Mixed Models in Medicine (Statistics in Practice)*. 2nd Edition, John Wiley & Sons Inc, Chichester.

Brown, P., and Ezekowitz, J. (2017). Power and sample size estimation for nonparametric composite endpoints: Practical implementation using data simulations. *Journal of Modern Applied Statistical Methods*, 16, 215–230.

Buyse, M. (2010). Generalized pairwise comparisons of prioritized outcomes in the two-sample problem. *Statistics in Medicine*, 29, 3245–3257.

Chen, C., Li, X., Yuan, S., Antonijevic, Z., Kalamegham, R., & Beckman, R. A. (2016). Statistical design and considerations of a phase 3 basket trial for simultaneous investigation of multiple tumor types in one study. *Statistics in Biopharmaceutical Research*, 8(3), 248–257.

Chen, Y. H. J, DeMets, D. L., & Lan, K. K. G. (2004). Increasing the sample size when the unblinded interim result is promising. *Statistics in Medicine*, 23(7), 1023–1038.

Chen, Y. J., Gesser, R., & Luxembourg, A. (2014). A seamless phase IIb/III adaptive outcome trial: Design rationale and implementation challenges. *Clinical Trials*, 12(1), 84–90.

Chow, S.-C., & Liu, J.-P. (2008). *Design and Analysis of Bioavailability and Bioequivalence Studies* (3rd ed.). Chapman and Hall/CRC. https://doi.org/10.1201/9781420011678

Chu, Y. & Yuan, Y. (2018). A Bayesian basket trial design using a calibrated bayesian hierarchical model. *Clinical Trials*, 15(2), 149–158.

Cohen, A., & Sackrowitz, H. B. (1989). Two stage conditionally unbiased estimators of the selected mean. *Statistics & Probability Letters*, 8, 273–278.

Conroy, S., Choonara, I., Impicciatore, P., Mohn, A., Arnell, H., Rane, A., . . . & van Den Ankar, J. (2000). Survey of unlicensed and off label drug use in paediatric wards in European countries. *British Medical Journal*, 320(7227): 79.

Cui, L., Hung, J. H. M., & Wang, S. J. (1999). Modification of sample size in group sequential clinical trials. *Biometrics*, 55(3), 853–857.

Cui, L., Zhan, T., Zhang, L., Geng, Z., Gu, Y., & Chan, I. S. (2021). An automation-based adaptive seamless design for dose selection and confirmation with improved power and efficiency. *Statistical Methods in Medical Research*, 30(4), 1013–1025.

Cunanan, K. M., Iasonos, A., Shen, R., Begg, C. B., & Gönen, M. (2017). An efficient basket trial design. *Statistics in Medicine*, 36(10), 1568–1579.

Dai, H., Leeder, J., & Cui, Y. (2014). A modified generalized Fisher method for combining probabilities from dependent tests. *Frontiers in Genetics*, 5, 32.

Dallow, N. S., Leonov, S. L., & Roger, J. H. (2008). Practical usage of O'Brien's OLS and GLS statistics in clinical trials. *Pharmaceutical Statistics*, 7, 53–68.

Davies, J. C., Wainwright, C. E., Canny, G. J., Chilvers, M. A., Howenstine, M. S., Munck, A., ... & Ahrens, R. (2013). Efficacy and safety of Ivacaftor in patients aged 6 to 11 years with cystic fibrosis with a G551D mutation. *American Journal of Respiratory and Critical Care Medicine, 187*(11), 1219–1225.

Deltuvaite-Thomas, V., & Burzykowski, T. (2021). Operational characteristics of generalized pairwise comparisons for hierarchically ordered endpoints. *Pharmaceutical Statistics, 21*(1), 122–132.

Diamond, E. L., Subbiah, V., Lockhart, C., Blay, J. Y., Faris, J. E., Puzanov, I., ... & Hyman, D. M. (2016). Vemurafenib in patients with Erdheim-Chester disease (ECD) and Langerhans cell histiocytosis (LCH) harboring BRAFV600 mutations: A cohort of the histology-independent VE-Basket study. *Blood, 128*(22), 480.

Dmitrienko, A., Tamhane, A. C., & Bretz, F. (2009). *Multiple Testing Problems in Pharmaceutical Statistics*, CRC Press, Boca Raton.

EMA/CHMP. (2006). Guideline on clinical trials in small populations. [Online]. [Cited: January 18, 2022]. https://www.ema.europa.eu/en/documents/scientific-guideline/guideline-clinical-trials-small-populations_en.pdf

European Medicines Agency, Committee for Medicinal Products for Human Use (Chmp). (2006). Guideline On Clinical Trials In Small Populations. https://www.ema.europa.eu/en/documents/scientific-guideline/guideline-clinical-trials-small-populations_en.pdf

Feingold, M., & Gillespie, B.W. (1996). Cross-over trials with censored data. *Statistics in Medicine, 15*(10), 953–967.

Finkelstein, D. M., & Schoenfeld, D. A. (1999). Combining mortality and longitudinal measures in clinical trials. *Statistics in Medicine, 18*, 1341–1354.

Fisher, R. A. (1925), *Statistical Methods for Research Workers*. Oliver and Boyd, Edinburgh.

Flaherty, K. R., Wells, A. U., Cottin, V., Devaraj, A., Walsh, S. L., Inoue, Y., ... & Brown, K. K. (2019). Nintedanib in progressive fibrosing interstitial lung diseases. *New England Journal of Medicine, 381*(18), 1718–1727.

Follmann, D. A., Proschan, M. A., & Geller, N. L. (1994). Monitoring pairwise comparisons in multi-armed clinical trials. *Biometrics, 50*, 325–336.

Freidlin, B., & Korn, E. L. (2014). Biomarker enrichment strategies: Matching trial design to biomarker credentials. *Nature Reviews Clinical Oncology, 11*, 81–90.

Freidlin, B., Sun, Z., Gray, R., & Korn, E. L. (2013). Phase III clinical trials that integrate treatment and biomarker evaluation. *Journal of Clinical Oncology, 31*, 3158–3161.

Friede, T., Parsons, N., Stallard, N., Todd, S., Valdes Marquez, E., Chataway, J., & Nicholas, R. (2011). Designing a seamless phase II/III clinical trial using early outcomes for treatment selection: An application in multiple sclerosis. *Statistics in Medicine, 30*(13), 1528–1540.

Gagne, J. J., Thompson, L., O'Keefe, K., & Kesselheim, A. S. (2014). Innovative research methods for studying treatments for rare diseases: Methodological review. *British Medical Journal, 349*, g6802.

Gallagher, J. R., Lapidus, D., Heap, K., & Carroll, S. (2019). Prevalence of Diagnosed/ Highly symptomatic pachyonychia congenita patients managed annually by US dermatologists – National Real World Occurrence (RWO) physician study. *Journal of Dermatology Disease, 6*, 280.

Gao, P., Ware, J. H., & Mehta, C. (2008). Sample size re-estimation for adaptive sequential design in clinical trials. *Journal of Biopharmaceutical Statistics, 18*(6), 1184–1196.

Gart, J. J. (1969). An exact test for comparing matched proportions in crossover designs. *Biometrika, 56*, 75–80.

Guenther, W. C. (1981). Sample size formulas for normal theory t-tests. *The American Statistician, 35*, 243–244.

Harmatz P, Whitley C. B., Wang R. Y., Bauer M., Song W., Haller C., and Kakkis E. (2018). A novel blind start study design to investigate vestronidase alfa for mucopolysaccharidosis VII, an lutra-rare genetic disease. *Molecular Genetics and Metabolism, 123*, 488–494.

Hilgers, R. D., König, F., Molenberghs, G., & Senn, S. (2016). Design and analysis of clinical trials for small rare disease populations. *Journal of Rare Diseases Research & Treatment, 1*(3), 53–60.

Hsiao, S. T., Liu, L., & Mehta, C. R. (2018). Optimal promising zone designs. *Biometrical Journal, 61*(5), 1175–1186.

Hu, C., Dignam, J. J. (2019). Biomarker-driven oncology clinical trials: Key design elements, types, features, and practical considerations. *JCO Precision Oncology, 1*, 1–12.

Huber, A. M., Tomlinson, G. A., Koren, G., Feldman, B. M. (2007). Amitriptyline to relieve pain in juvenile idiopathic arthritis: a pilot study using Bayesian meta-analysis of multiple N-of-1 clinical trials. *Journal of Rheumatology, 34*(5), 1125–32.

Hughes, R., Donofrio, P., Bril, V., Dalakas, M. C., Deng, C., Hanna, K., ... & ICE Study Group. (2008). Intravenous immune globulin (10% caprylate-chromatography purified) for the treatment of chronic inflammatory demyelinating polyradiculoneuropathy (ICE Study): A randomised placebo-controlled trial. *Lancet Neurology. 7.* 136–44.

Hyman, D. M., Puzanov, I., Subbiah, V., Faris, J. E., Chau, I., Blay, J. Y., ... & Baselga, J. (2015). Vemurafenib in multiple nonmelanoma cancers with BRAF V600 mutations. *New England Journal of Medicine, 373*, 726–736.

IGIVnet Product Monograph (2019). https://www.grifols.com/documents/89713601/0/IGIVnex+-+English+PM+-+2017-07-12.pdf/98eb0376-0d61-491a-9fda-713505c61379

Inoue, L. Y., Thall, P. F., & Berry, D. A. (2002). Seamlessly expanding a randomized phase II trial to phase III. *Biometrics, 58*(4), 823–831.

James, N. D., Sydes, M. R., Clarke, N. W., Mason, M. D., Dearnaley, D. P., Spears, M. R., ... & de Bono, J. (2016). Addition of docetaxel, zoledronic acid, or both to first-line long-term hormone therapy in prostate cancer (STAMPEDE): Survival results from an adaptive, multiarm, multistage, platform randomised controlled trial. *The Lancet, 387*(10024), 1163–1177.

Jazić, I., Liu, X., & Laird, G. (2021). Design and analysis of drop-the-losers studies using binary endpoints in the rare disease setting. *Journal of Biopharmaceutical Statistics, 31*(4), 507–522.

Jenkins, M., Stone, A., Jennison, C. J. (2010). An adaptive seamless phase II/III design for oncology trials with subpopulation selection using correlated survival endpoints. *Pharmaceutical Statistics.* On-line version, DOI: 10.1002/pst.472.

Jennison, C., & Turnbull, B. W. (2000). *Group Sequential Methods with Applications to Clinical Trials.* Chapman and Hall/CRC, London.

Jennison, C., & Turnbull, B. W. (2015). Adaptive sample size modification in clinical trials: start small then ask for more? *Statistics in Medicine, 34*(29), 3793–3810.

Jones, B., & Kenward, M. G. (2014). *Design and Analysis of Cross-Over Trials,* 3rd Edition. Chapman and Hall, London.

Jones, R. L., Ravi, V., Brohl, A. S., Chawla, S. P., Ganjoo, K., Italiano, A., ... & Maki, R. (2019). Results of the TAPPAS trial: An adaptive enrichment phase III trial of TRC105 and pazopanib (P) versus pazopanib alone in patients with advanced angiosarcoma (AS). *Annals of Oncology*, 30 (Supplement 5), v683–v709.

Kelly, P. J., Stallard, N., & Todd, S. (2005). An adaptive group sequential design for phase II/III clinical trials that select a single treatment from several. *Journal of Biopharmaceutical Statistics*, 15(4), 641–658.

Kempf, L,. (2018). FDA Perspective on Clinical Trial Design for Rare Diseases, American Statistical Association Biopharm Workshop Sept, 2018.

Kenward, M. G., & Roger, J. H. (1997). Small sample inference for fixed effects from restricted maximum likelihood. Biometrics, 53(3), 983–997.

Kimani, P. K., Todd, S., & Stallard, N. (2014). A comparison of methods for constructing confidence intervals after phase II/III clinical trials. *Biometrical Journal*, 56(1), 107–128.

Koenig, F., Brannath, W., Bretz, F., & Posch, M. (2008). Adaptive Dunnett tests for treatment selection. *Statistics in Medicine*, 27, 1612–1625.

Korn, E. L., McShane, L. M., & Freidlin, B. (2013). Statistical challenges in the evaluation of treatments for small patient populations. *Science Translational Medicine*, 5(178):178sr3. doi: 10.1126/scitranslmed.3004018. PMID: 23536014.

Kotecha, M., Cheshire, W. P., Finnigan, H., Giblin, K., Naik, H., Palmer, J., ... & Zakrzewska, J. M. (2020). Design of phase 3 studies evaluating vixotrigine for treatment of trigeminal neuralgia. *Journal of Pain Research*, 13, 1601–1609.

Kunz, C. U., Friede, T., Parsons, N., Todd, S., & Stallard, N. (2014). Data-driven treatment selection for seamless phase II/III trials incorporating early-outcome data. *Pharmaceutical Statistics*, 13, 238–246.

Lan, K. K. G., & DeMets, D. L. (1983). Discrete sequential boundaries for clinical trials. Biometrika, 70(3):659–663.

Lancaster, H. O. (1961). The combination of probabilities: An application of orthonormal functions. *Australian Journal of Statistics*, 3(1), 20–33.

Langhlin, R. S., Dyck, P. J., Melton, L. J., Leibson, C., Ransom, J., & Dyck, P. J. B. (2009). Incidence and prevalence of CIDP and the association of diabetes mellitus. *Neurology*, 73(1), 39–45.

Lehmacher, W. & Wassmer, G. (1999). Adaptive sample size calculations in group sequential trials. *Biometrics*, 55, 1286–1290.

Logan, B. R., and Tamhane, A. C. (2004). On O'Brien's OLS and GLStests for multiple endpoints. *Recent Developments in Multiple Comparison Procedures*, 47, 76–88.

Lui, K. J., Chang, K. C. (2015). Sample size determination for testing nonequality under a three-treatment two-period incomplete block crossover trial. *Biometrical Journal*, 57(3), 410–21.

Mehrotra, D. V. (2014). A recommended analysis for 2 × 2 crossover trials with baseline measurements. *Pharmaceutical Statistics*, 13, 376–387.

Mehta, C. R., Liu, L., & Theuer, C. (2019). An adaptive population enrichment phase III trial of TRC105 and pazopanib versus pazopanib alone in patients with advanced angiosarcoma (TAPPAS trial). *Annals of Oncology*, 30(1), 103–108

Mehta, C. R., & Pocock, S. J. (2011). Adaptive increase in sample size when interim results arepromising: A practical guide with examples. *Statistics in Medicine*, 30(28), 3267–3284.

Miller, T., Cudkowicz, M., Shaw, P. J., Andersen, P. M., Atassi, N., Bucelli, R. C., ... & Ferguson, T. A. (2020). Phase 1–2 trial of antisense oligonucleotide tofersen for SOD1 ALS. *New England Journal of Medicine*, 383(2), 109–119.

Müller, H. H., & Schäfer, H. (2001). Adaptive group sequential designs for clinical trials: Combining the advantages of adaptive and of classical group sequential approaches. *Biometrics, 57*(3):886–891.

Nikles, J., Mitchell, G., McKinlay, L., Waugh, M.-C., Epps, A., Carmont, S.-A., Schluter, P.J., Lloyd, O., & Senior, H. (2017). A series of n-of-1 trials of stimulants in brain injured children. *NeuroRehabilitation, 40,* 11–21.

O'Brien, P. C. (1984). Procedures for comparing samples with multiple endpoints. *Biometrics, 40,* 1079–1087.

Palvella Therapeutics. (2020). Palvella Therapeutics Reports Top-Line Results from Pivotal Phase 2/3 VALO Trial of QTORIN™ 3.9% Rapamycin Anhydrous Gel in Patients with Pachyonychia Congenita. https://palvellatx.com/2020/12/23/palvella-thera-peutics-reports-top-line-results-from-pivotal-phase-2-3-valo-trial-of-qtorin-3-9-ra-pamycin-anhydrous-gel-in-patients-with-pachyonychia-congenita/

Park, J. W., Liu, M. C., Yee, D., Yau, C., van't Veer, L. J., Symmans, W. F., ... & DeMichele, A. (2016). Adaptive randomization of neratinib in early breast cancer. *New England Journal of Medicine, 375*(1), 11–22.

Pocock, S. J., Ariti, C. A., Collier, T. J., & Wang, D. (2012). The win ratio: A new approach to the analysis of composite endpoints in clinical trials based on clinical priori-ties. *European Heart Journal, 33,* 176–182.

Pocock, S. J., Geller, N. L., & Tsiatis, A. A. (1987). The analysis of multiple endpoints in clinical trials. *Biometrics, 43,* 487–498.

Posch, M., Koenig, F., Branson, M., Brannath, W., Dunger-Baldauf, C., & Bauer, P. (2005). Testing and estimation in flexible group sequential designs with adap-tive treatment selection. *Statistics in Medicine, 24,* 3697–3714.

Prentice, R. L. (1989). Surrogate endpoints in clinical trials: Defintion and operational criteria. *Statistics in Medicine, 8,* 431–440.

Prescott, R. J. (1981). The comparison of success rates in cross-over trials in the pres-ence of an order effect. *Applied Statistics, 30,* 9–15

Quan, H., Luo, X., Zhou, T., & Zhao, P.-L. (2020). Seamless phase II/III/IIIb clinical trial designs with different endpoints for different phases. *Communications in Statistics - Theory and Methods, 49*(22), 5436–5454.

Quan, H., Xu, Y., Chen, Y., Gao, L., & Chen, X. (2018). A case study of an adaptive design for a clinical trial with 2 doses and 2 endpoints in a rare disease area. *Pharmaceutical Statistics, 17,* 797–810.

Ramsey, B. W., Davies, J., McElvaney, N. G., Tullis, E., Bell, S. C., Dřevínek, P., ... & Elborn, J. S. (2011). A CFTR potentiator in patients with cystic fibrosis and the G551D mutation. *New England Journal of Medicine, 365,* 1663–1672.

Ristl, R., Urach, S., Rosenkranz, G., & Posch, M. (2019). Methods for the analysis of multiple endpoints in small populations: A review. *Journal of Biopharmaceutical Statistics, 29,* 1–29.

Sampson, A. R., & Sill, M. W. (2005). Drop-the-losers design: Normal case. *Biometrical Journal, 47*(3), 257–268.

Schaid, D. J., Wieand, S., & Therneau, T. M. (1990). Optimal two-stage screening designs for survival comparisons. *Biometrika, 77*(3), 507–513.

Scharfstein, D. O., Tsiatis, A.A., & Robins, J .M. (1997). Semiparametric efficiency and its implication on the design and analysis of group-sequential studies. *Journal of the American Statistical Association, 92,* 1342–1350.

Schultz, J. R., Nichol, F. R., Elfring, G. L. & Weed, S. D. (1973). Multiple-stage proce-dures for drug screening. *Biopharmaceutics, 15,* 657–680.

Senn, S. (2002). *Cross-Over Trials in Clinical Research.* Wiley, Chichester.

Senn, S., & Bretz, F. (2007). Power and sample size when multiple endpoints are considered. *Pharmaceutical Statistics: The Journal of Applied Statistics in the Pharmaceutical Industry, 6*, 161–170.

Shaffer, J. A., Falzon, L., Cheung, K., Davidson, K. W. (2015). N-of-1 randomized trials for psychological and health behavior outcomes: A systematic review protocol. *Systematic Reviews, 4*, 87.

Sheehe, P. R., & Bross, I. D. J. (1961). Latin squares to balance immediate residual and other effects. *Biometrics, 17*, 405–414.

Sill, M. W., & Sampson, A. R. (2009). Drop-the-losers design: Binomial case. *Computational Statistics and Data Analysis, 53*, 586–595.

Simon, R. (1989). Optimal two-stage designs for phase II clinical trials. *Controlled Clinical Trials, 10*(1), 1–10.

Simon, R., Geyer, S., Subramanian, J., & Roychowdhury, S. (2016). The Bayesian basket design for genomic variant-driven phase II trials. *Seminars in Oncology, 43*(1), 13–18.

Stallard, N. (2010). A confirmatory seamless phase II/III clinical trial design incorporating short-term endpoint information. *Statistics in Medicine, 29*, 959–971.

Stallard, N., & Todd, S. (2003). Sequential designs for phase III clinical trials incorporating treatment selection. *Statistics in Medicine, 22*, 689–703.

Stokes, M. E., Davis, C. S., & Koch, G. G. (2012). *Categorical Data Analysis Using the SAS System*, 3rd Edition, SAS Institute Inc., Cary, NC.

Stouffer, S. A., Suchman, E. A., DeVinney, L. C., Star, S. A., & Williams Jr, R. M. (1949). *The American Soldier: Adjustment during Army Life. (Studies in Social Psychology in World War II)*, vol. 1, Princeton University Press, Princeton.

Stroup, W. W. (2012). *Generalized Linear Mixed Models: Modern Concepts, Methods and Applications*. CRC Press, Boca Raton.

Stunnenberg, B. C., Woertman, W., Raaphorst, J., Statland, J. M., Griggs, R., Timmermans, J., Saris, C. G., Schouwenberg, B. J., Groenewoud, H. M., Stegeman, D. F., Engelen, B., Drost, G., Wilt, G. (2015). Combined N-of-1 trials to investigate mexiletine in non-dystrophic myotonia using a Bayesian approach; study rationale and protocol. *BMC Neurology, 15*, 43.

Sun, H., Davison, B. A., Cotter, G., Pencina, M. J., & Koch, G. G. (2012). Evaluating treatment efficacy by multiple end points in phase II acute heart failure clinical trials: Analyzing data using a global method, *Circulation: Heart Failure, 5*, 742–749.

Sung, L., Tomlinson, G. A., Greenberg, M. L., Koren, G., Judd, P., Ota, S., Feldman, B. M. (2007). Serial controlled N-of-1 trials of topical vitamin E as prophylaxis for chemotherapy-induced oral mucositis in paediatric patients. *European Journal of Cancer, 43*, 1269–1275.

Tappin, L. (1992). Unbiased estimation of the parameter of a selected binomial population. *Communications in Statistics - Theory and Methods, 21*(4), 1067–1083.

Tardivon, C., Desmee, S., Kerioui, M., Bruno, R., Wu, B., Mentre, F., ... & Guedj, J. (2019). Association between tumor size kinetics and survivals in patients with urothelial carcinoma treated with atezolizumab implication for patient follow-up. *Clinical Pharmacology & Therapeutics, 106*, 810–820.

Thall, P. (2021). Adaptive enrichment designs in clinical trials. *Annual Review of Statistics and Its Application, 8*, 393–411.

Thall, P. F., Simon, R., & Ellenberg, S. S. (1988). Two-stage selection and testing designs for comparative clinical trials. *Biometrika, 75*(2), 303–310.

Thall, P. F., Simon, R., & Ellenberg, S. S. (1989). A two-stage design for choosing among several experimental treatments and a control in clinical trials. *Biometrics, 45*(2), 537–547.

Thall, P. F., Wathen, J. K., Bekele, B. N., Champlin, R. E., Baker, L. H., & Benjamin, R. S. (2003). Hierarchical Bayesian approaches to phase II trials in diseases with multiple subtypes. *Statistics in Medicine, 22,* 763–780.

The White House (2015). Remarks by the President in State of the Union Address. Available from: https://obamawhitehouse.archives.gov/the-press-office/2015/01/20/remarks-president-state-union-address-January-20-2015. Access on 25 Jun 2019.

Todd, S., & Stallard, N. (2005). A new clinical trial design combining phases 2 and 3: Sequential designs with treatment selection and a change of endpoint. *Drug Information Journal, 39,* 109–118.

Tudor, G., & Koch, G. G. (1994). Review of nonparametric methods for the analysis of crossover studies. *Statistical Methods in Medical Research, 3,* 345–381.

U.S. Food and Drug Administration (2018). *Developing Targeted Therapies in Low-Frequency Molecular Subsets of a Disease,* US FDA, Rockville, MD.

U.S. Food and Drug Administration (2019a). *Draft Guidance, Rare Diseases: Common Issues in Drug Development Guidance for Industry,* US FDA, Rockville, MD.

U.S. Food and Drug Administration (2019b). *Guidance for Industry: Enrichment Strategies for Clinical Trials to Support Approval of Human Drugs and Biological Products.*

Valeyre, D., Duchemann, B., Nunes, H., Uzunhan, Y., & Annesi-Maesano, I. (2014). Interstitial lung diseases. *Respiratory Epidemiology.* Chapter 6, Vol. 65, 79–87.

Wang, S.-J., O'Neill, R. T., & Hung, H. M. J. (2007). Approaches to evaluation of treatment effect in randomized clinical trials with genomic subset. *Pharmaceutical Statistics, 6*(3):227–44.

Wason, J. M., & Jaki, T. (2012). Optimal design of multi-arm multi-stage trials. *Statistics in Medicine, 31*(30), 4269–4279.

Wason, J. M., & Trippa, L. (2014). A comparison of Bayesian adaptive randomization and multi-stage designs for multi-arm clinical trials. *Statistics in Medicine, 33*(13), 2206–2221.

Wason, J., Stallard, N., Bowden, J., & Jennison, C. (2017). A multi-stage drop-the-losers design for multi-arm clinical trials. *Statistical Methods in Medical Research, 26*(1), 508–524.

Wathen, J. K., Thall, P. F., Cook, J. D., & Estey, E. H. (2008). Accounting for patient heterogeneity in phase II clinical trials. *Statistics in Medicine, 27*(15): 2802–2815.

Williams, E. J. (1949). Experimental designs balanced for the estimation of residual effects of treatments. *Australian Journal of Chemistry, 2,* 149–168.

Woodcock, J., & LaVange, L. M. (2017). Master protocols to study multiple therapies, multiple diseases, or both. *New England Journal of Medicine, 377*(1), 62–70.

Yap, C., & Cheung, Y. K. (2018). Sequential elimination in multi-arm multi-stage selection trials. In *Wiley StatsRef: Statistics Reference Online.* https://onlinelibrary.wiley.com/doi/book/10.1002/9781118445112

Zakrzewska, J. M., Palmer, J., Morisset, V., Giblin, G. M., Obermann, M., Ettlin, D. A., ... & Tate S. (2017). Safety and efficacy of a Nav1.7 selective sodium channel blocker in patients with trigeminal neuralgia: A double-blind, placebo-controlled, randomised withdrawal phase 2a trial. *The Lancet Neurology, 16*(4, 291–300.

Zaykin, D. V., Zhivotovsky, L. A., Westfall, P. H., & Weir, B. S. (2002). Truncated product method for combining P-values. *Genetic Epidemiology, 22,* 170–185.

Zhan, T., Cui, L., Geng, Z., Zhang, L., Gu, Y., & Chan, I. S. (2021). A practical response adaptive block randomization (RABR) design with analytic type I error protection. *Statistics in Medicine, 40*(23), 4947–4960.

Zhu, H., Piao, J., Lee, J. J., Hu, F., & Zhang, L. (2020). Response adaptive randomization procedures in seamless phase II/III clinical trials. *Journal of Biopharmaceutical Statistics, 30*(1), 3–17.

Zucker, D. R., Ruthazer, R., Schmid, C. H. (2010). Individual (N-of-1) trials can be combined to give population comparative treatment effect estimates: methodologic considerations. *Journal of Clinical Epidemiology, 63* (12), 1312–1323.

5

Use of Real-World Evidence to Support Drug Development

Lina Titievsky and Nataliya Volkova

Vertex Pharmaceuticals

CONTENTS

DOI: 10.1201/9781003080954-5

5.1 Introduction: Value of RWE across the Rare Disease Drug Development Stages

Real-world evidence (RWE) generated using real-world data (RWD) is an integral component of drug development. In this chapter, we discuss the uses of RWE across different stages of drug development in support of rare disease therapies. We start by defining RWD and RWE and their uses across drug development stages, and we then proceed to discuss the types of RWD sources that researchers can consider in studying rare diseases and conclude by focusing on practicalities and challenges in generating the right type of RWE at each of these stages of rare disease drug development. While many concepts discussed here also apply to the use of RWE in support of market access and reimbursement, these uses are not discussed here.

5.1.1 RWD and RWE Definitions

Both the European Medicines Agency (EMA) and the US Food and Drug Administration (FDA) use "routinely collected" as the underlying definition of real-world data (RWD):

> routinely collected data of a patient's health status or the delivery of health care from a variety of sources' that is beyond conventional clinical trials, including electronic health records (EHRs), claims, registries, patient-generated data, and other data sources that can generate health status, such as mobile devices.[1,2]

RWE, in turn, is the clinical evidence that is derived from the analysis of RWD. RWE can be generated by different study designs or analyses, including but not limited to pragmatic trials and observational studies (prospective and/or retrospective).

While there is an increasing recognition in the value of RWD and RWE, their use to support regulatory decision-making is not a new phenomenon and RWD have been used for over 30 years for safety signal evaluation, risk management, and benefit–risk evaluation.[1,3] Both FDA and EMA have been extensively using real-world databases for signal surveillance and assessment.[4-6] Although there has been a lower acceptability of RWE for assessment of efficacy/effectiveness with preference given to randomized control trials (RCTs) as a gold standard for evidence generation, the rapid pace of change in the scientific and technological landscapes, which include adoption of digital technologies and increasing sources of new data source, may increase the regulatory acceptability of RWE use for effectiveness as well. Importantly, traditional drug development pathway may not be suitable for all therapies such as advanced therapies or orphan products for conditions with significant unmet need and for which a traditional RCT may be unfeasible or unethical resulting in single-arm clinical studies.[7]

5.1.2 Role of RWE across the Lifecycle of Rare Disease Drug Development

RWE plays an important role starting from the very early stages of rare disease drug development. As early as preclinical stage, RWE can be effectively used to quantify the size (e.g., prevalence) of the potential target patient population, evaluate burden of illness and unmet medical need, and study the natural history of disease. Across all drug development stages, RWE can generate useful insights about the background occurrence of events of interest (both efficacy markers and potential safety concerns) in the target populations of patients which can in turn contextualize the accruing clinical trial data. Finally, in the post-authorization stage, RWE is essential to evaluate the effects of medicines under the real-world conditions of use, including post-marketing safety monitoring and effectiveness evaluations, and may also be used to support product label expansions. The figure below illustrates the role that RWE plays in early drug development, later drug development, and post-authorization stages (Figure 5.1).

5.2 RWD Collection Approaches in Rare Disease Research

Until recently, two main sources of RWD have included – primary data (data collected in the real-world setting "de novo," i.e., specifically for the study) and secondary use of data (existing data that had been already collected for another purpose). However, with the adoption of technology and increased opportunities for data linkage, an enriched study method can be used which enables linking primary and secondary data. Methodological

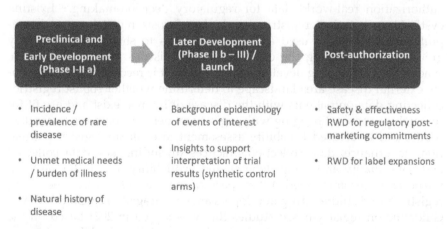

FIGURE 5.1
Role of RWE across drug development life cycle.

considerations are discussed in a number of guidance documents and peer-reviewed publications.[8-10]

Rare disease research is not an exception and may rely on either primary data collection or secondary use of data. There is no "one size fits all" strategy that can be recommended for all rare disease studies utilizing RWD. The decision on the choice of the optimal study design and data source(s) is made after research questions have been clearly formulated following a careful feasibility assessment of all available data collection options. Below, we focus our e-discussion on select high-level considerations and principles for real-world data collection approaches for rare disease drug development.

5.2.1 Secondary Use of Data Collected by Existing Rare Disease Registries

Patient registries are defined as organized data collection systems gathering uniform data to identify specified outcomes for a population defined by a particular disease, condition, or exposure. Consequently, rare disease registries are registries whose members are defined by a particular rare disease, regardless of their exposure to any medicinal product, other treatment, or health service.[11,12]

Robust existing rare disease registries can be an invaluable source of data for orphan drug development, and their use can be encouraged or even requested by regulators in the context of either pre-approval natural history data needs or post-approval safety and effectiveness evaluations.

Regulators are invested in maximizing the use of disease registries in drug development. Most recently, EMA launched a Registry Initiative to optimize the use of existing registries and/or facilitate the establishment of high-quality new registries to provide an adequate source of post-authorization real-world data for regulatory decision-making.[13] Existing cystic fibrosis patient registries, multiple sclerosis registries, and hemophilia registries were used as model registries to shape EMA's registry guidance, emphasizing the critical role of registries in the rare disease space. Early in the drug development program, it is recommended to evaluate external disease area landscape to determine whether robust registries collecting data on patients with the disease of interest exist and are fit for research purposes. Engaging with registry owners or operators to conduct robust and structured feasibility assessment to evaluate registry population, governance, data collection practices (including key data collected and data quality and completeness), and availability of data for research purposes is recommended. When performing feasibility assessments for registry-based studies, drug developers are encouraged to consult the EMA Guideline on registry-based studies that was issued in 2021 based on the Registry Initiative efforts, and which addresses the methodological, regulatory, and operational aspects involved in using registry-based studies to support regulatory decision-making.[11] Similar, more recent guideline from FDA should also be consulted.[14] Other useful resources include EMA Registry Initiative website[15] and the ENCePP Resources database[16] serving as a repository of RWD sources, including rare disease registries. There are examples of successful use of patient registries to support rare disease drug development. For instance, cystic fibrosis (CF) patient registries have been successfully used to support drug development of CFTR modulators.

5.2.2 Secondary Use of Healthcare Record Databases and Multi-Database Studies

Electronic administrative data sources, including claims and electronic medical records have a long history of being used as a data source for generating RWE in drug development, with key principles covered in regulatory guidance documents, such as FDA Use of Electronic Health Record Data in Clinical Investigations Guidance for Industry.[17] Claims data consist of the billing codes that different providers submit to payers and enable a holistic view of the patient's interaction with the health care system. EHR systems are electronic platforms that contain individual health records for patients. The extent to which one's EHR reflects all encounters with the healthcare systems varies by country. While both claims and EHR provide data on a large number of patients, none of these data sources has been designed in mind for research. As such, it is important to carefully evaluate the potential use administrative data source to generate RWE in support of rare diseases based on the following considerations:

1. It may or may not be possible to precisely identify patients with rare disease of interest in EHRs as the coverage of International Classification of Disease (ICD) for rare diseases is not universal. For instance, it has been estimated out of approximately 6,500 rare diseases, only about 11% have available corresponding ICD-9-CM codes and about 21% with ICD-10 codes.[18] This lack of codes may pose a significant barrier for using electronic administrative data sources for rare disease RWE generation.

2. Electronic administrative data sources lack the clinical depth necessary to address a particular research objective in a rare disease of interest. For instance, for genetic conditions, genotype information may be either completely lacking or not available in a structured form in many available healthcare record databases. Additionally, disease severity or patient characteristics requiring access to laboratory and/or imaging results may not be available for all patients. Natural language processing (NLP) techniques have been increasingly leveraged in some cases to overcome this challenge by accessing

unstructured data in clinical notes as a source of additional clinical details.[19]

3. In the case of rare diseases, one data source may have an insufficient coverage of the target patient population and/or size of the patient population insufficient for robust evaluation of research question of interest. Multi-database studies (MDSs) may offer a potential solution to maximize the population coverage and study size. A MDS uses at least two healthcare databases, which are not linked with each other at an individual person level, with analyses carried out in parallel across each database applying a common study protocol.[20]

5.2.3 Primary Data Collection

If it is not possible to identify an appropriate existing registry or administrative data source with relevant clinical detail and/or adequate number of patients with rare disease of interest, prospective primary data collection to address research objectives may be considered. Primary data collection studies may include stand-alone cohort studies or de novo registries. However, these represent a significant resource and operational burden and, therefore, should be carefully planned, including but not limited to the following steps:

1. Thorough feasibility assessment is imperative in planning of the primary data collection studies. The questions that should be addressed include whether there is interest and support for the initiation of de novo study from patients and external scientific community and whether there are any competing ongoing studies or research efforts (e.g., resource-consuming clinical trials or observational studies). Patient advocacy groups play an important role in providing critical insights in this process. Feasibility assessment should include desired geographies and number of potential study sites resulting in an outreach to the potential participating sites initiated. Site assessment needs to address site interest to participate or factors limiting participation, prior experience with research study conduct, size of patient population seen at the site, and ability to comply with the study protocol, including required data collection and any adverse event reporting requirements.

2. As any primary data collection is associated with considerable resource requirements, a thoughtful approach to data collection is warranted in order to balance the need for high quality of data with the volume to address the research question(s) while considering the site burden.

5.3 RWE in Early Stages of Drug Development for Rare Disease

At the early stages of drug development, real-world data are used to understand the size and geographic distribution of the patient population along with the unmet medical need and natural history of the rare disease of interest.

5.3.1 Quantifying Target Patient Population

Epidemiology data are often used to estimate the size of the target population, quantify and describe demographic and clinical characteristics, and help determine the potential public health impact that the therapy will have once it is marketed and prescribed to the general population.[21] Point prevalence is typically the most appropriate measure of the population burden of disease in the case of rare diseases (i.e., number of affected individuals with a disease under consideration). One of the major advantages of point prevalence is that it is not influenced by the length of the study period and consequently is not impacted by mortality or migration as other measures of disease frequency (e.g., birth prevalence).[22] Point prevalence plays a critical role in the current orphan drug legislation where definition of rare diseases includes a prevalence-based threshold.[23] Obtaining prevalence estimates for rare diseases from published literature and/or quantifying prevalence estimates from available data sources is often challenging. This is because as pointed out in Sections 5.2.1 and 5.2.2, some diseases may be poorly characterized in literature and/or no standard definition for a given disease exits and/or, if a definition exists, there are limited data sources that capture information on that disease in a consistent manner. In those circumstances where a rare disease can be identified via ICD-10 codes and/or NLPs, it is possible to apply machine learning to improve patient identification.

Given the shift toward a precision medicine, a new therapy targets only a sub-sample of patients with a rare disease, and it is not unusual to have limited published data on this sub-population as there has been no prior scientific incentive to examine this disease in the absence of potential treatment(s). Consequently, it is often necessary to rely on the diversity of the data, with none of the sources being optimal, which are derived from a variety of disparate information sources that include literature reviews, patient registries, published case series, expert opinions, and other anecdotal evidence. This is complicated by the need to account for country-specific differences. Since many rare diseases have a genetic basis, it is not always possible to generalize findings from one country to another because the distribution of genetic variants may differ. Further, in the context of rare diseases, it is relevant to consider the role of migration and its effect on disease distribution and prevalence.

It is necessary to critically appraise available literature whenever using published literature when estimating the prevalence of rare diseases. To our knowledge, no checklists for the assessment of methodological quality of rare disease studies are available today. While the Strengthening the Reporting of Observational Studies in Epidemiology (STROBE) guidelines[24] is a useful tool for observational studies in general, these do not appear to be the most suitable tool for assessing the quality of prevalence studies in rare diseases as these guidelines do not account for the variable sources from which prevalence data may be ascertained or include relevant considerations for the prevalence studies in rare diseases such as consanguinity, ethnicity, etc.[22] Based on one of the few systematic literature reviews aimed at quantifying prevalence of a rare disease with an in-depth assessment of each study quality, it was highlighted that there is an appreciable amount of misunderstanding regarding how prevalence data should be reported and that various measures of disease were used interchangeably (i.e., incidence, prevalence, frequency, and birth prevalence).[22] Using different measures of disease interchangeably will lead to flawed and inaccurate estimates. Additionally, depending on a study methodology (e.g., specifics of a disease definition, limiting to certain regions of the country, use of referral centers), it is possible to under- and overestimate prevalence. When presenting estimates of prevalence estimates, it is important to be transparent in the methods and data sources used, and any assumptions made.

5.3.2 Evaluating Burden of Illness/Natural History of Disease

The natural history of a disease is defined as the course a disease takes in the absence of intervention in individuals with the disease, from the time of onset until either resolution or death.[7] A natural history study is a pre-planned observational study aimed at identifying demographic, genetic, environment, and other relevant variable that correlated with the disease development and outcomes.

There are various potential uses of a natural history study across all phases of drug development for rare diseases. FDA's Draft Guidance for Industry "Rare Diseases: Natural History Studies for Drug Development"[7] provides a comprehensive review of the four key uses of natural history studies during drug development: (1) identifying the patient population for a particular therapy; (2) identification or development of clinical outcomes assessments; (3) identification or development of biomarkers; and (4) design of externally controlled studies. For example, much of what is known about the natural history of Gaucher disease is a consequence of establishing International Collaborative Gaucher Group (ICGG) Gaucher Registry. ICGG is a global initiative that has enrolled more than 6,000 patients with longitudinal data collection on disease severity, quality of life, age of presentation, and therapeutic responses. Prior to the establishment of this registry, much of what was known about Gaucher disease was based on small case series or isolated case reports. This registry has served as a platform for collaboration and a large number of registry-based studies resulting in key insights including delineation of the phenotypic spectrum in children with Gaucher disease (GD) type 1 and providing evidence into the pediatric onset of GD type 1. Additional findings included understanding the expected course of disease such as increased risk of cancer and Parkinson's disease, course of skeletal disease among patients, and impact of splenectomy on the natural history. These findings in turn have shaped treatment guidelines for GD, established benchmark (aka background) rates of various complications of disease, and informed clinical trial design such as endpoints selection, duration of follow-up, and sample size estimations.[25]

No one rare disease is the same, and as such, natural history study design characteristics, data sources, and study methods all require a careful assessment through the "fit-for-purpose" lens. Much of the approach in Sections 5.2.1 and 5.2.2 is applicable here.

5.4 RWE in Later Stages of Drug Development for Rare Disease

5.4.1 RWE as an External Control Arm

Given the number of single-arm clinical studies in rare diseases, an externally controlled trial warrants a consideration. An externally controlled trial is one which the control group consists of patients who are not part of the same randomized study as the group receiving the investigational agent; that is, there is no concurrently randomized control group".[26] Use of external controls is acceptable under select circumstances such as diseases with high and predictable mortality or progressive morbidity or when it is not feasible or ethical to use an "internal control" and/or when a state of clinical equipoise may not exist.[27] The use of an external control group may be necessary with either single-arm trials or uncontrolled long-term extension studies (LTE). In contrast to an internal control group that is drawn from the same population, an external control is a group of patients that is external to the study.[28] External controls can be broadly divided into historical or concurrent controls. RWE generated from external controls can serve as real-world benchmarks (rather than as "formal" comparators) or as real-world comparators[7,26–29] which is determined by the regulatory and clinical context. Typically, real-world benchmark data are used for contextualization, whereas real-world "formal" comparators require a more stringent application which includes mirroring the patient population via application of the same inclusion and exclusion criteria along with the analytical techniques such as propensity score matching and formal analyses of the external comparator population to that of the trial.[26–29] Externally controlled trials have been gaining regulatory acceptance in rare diseases because many clinical trials are conducted with very few patients and hence low statistical power or are performed as single-arm trials.[27] Various examples of external controls are presented in Chapter 8.

5.4.2 RWE to Contextualize Potential Safety Concerns Arising during the Course of Rare Disease Product Development

As previously discussed in Chapter 2, rare disease clinical development programs are likely to include relatively small numbers of patients and randomization may not be feasible or ethical, leaving single-arm trial design as the only option. Consequently, it may be challenging to interpret whether potential adverse events arising during the course of such development programs, in particular rare or uncommon events, are causally related to investigational therapies. Regulatory-grade RWE describing the occurrence of such events of interest in the indicated disease or condition is an important tool for the sponsors and regulators to differentiate potential safety concerns from the events inherent to the disease or condition itself.

The ability to estimate and characterize a background risk using real-world data enables to assess potentials safety signals using expected versus observed analyses and complement other ongoing pharmacovigilance efforts.

5.5 RWE for Post-Marketing Safety and Effectiveness Evaluations of Rare Disease Therapies

Clinical trial data package at the time or regulatory approval may be limited, including small patient population, short follow-up, approval obtained based on a surrogate endpoint, and in some cases absence of control arm. For these reasons, post-marketing evaluation of key safety and effectiveness outcomes, as well as drug utilization patterns under the real-world conditions of use bridges important evidence gaps and is of particular interest to sponsors, regulators, payers and rare disease patients and research community.

These post-marketing safety and effectiveness evaluations may be initiated, managed or financed by drug developers either voluntarily or as an obligation imposed by regulatory agencies. Applicable regulatory guidelines should be followed when planning and implementing real-world post-marketing safety and effectiveness studies, including but not limited to EMA Scientific Guidance on Post-Authorisation Efficacy Studies, EMA Guideline on Good Pharmacovigilance Practices: Module VIII – Post-Authorisation Safety Studies, and FDA Guidance for Industry: Post-marketing Studies and Clinical Trials.

General observational research principles and good practices apply to post-marketing safety and effectiveness evaluations in rare disease; however, the following challenges should be noted:

1. Sample size of the post-marketing study will be dependent on the product uptake and utilization in the real world setting and may be limited and insufficient for robust statistical analyses in rare diseases. Researchers may consider multi-national studies, studies with longer patient accrual or enrollment periods, or both to maximize the evaluable patient population.

2. Identification of concurrent untreated comparator population may represent a challenge in rare disease, in particular when the new therapy under study has a high uptake rate. Researchers may need to evaluate alternative comparator approaches, such as external historical comparator from a calendar period preceding availability of the therapy of interest, untreated comparator population from a different geographic area where therapy of interest is not available yet, proxy concurrent comparator population (e.g., patients of different genotype but similar phenotype to indicated patient population), or all of these approaches combined.

3. Certain rare disease therapies may require very long follow-up in the real-world setting, which may present a challenge. For instance, regulatory agencies mandate 15-year follow-up of patients receiving gene editing therapies. Researchers need to maximize data completeness and quality while minimizing patient loss to follow-up over such long time periods.

Despite these challenges, post-marketing safety and effectiveness evaluations of rare disease therapies are invaluable to supplement trial data and generate evidence under the real-world conditions of use.

5.6 RWE for Label Expansions

There is an increasing number of examples of label expansion using RWE. This is usually done when a drug is already on the market, and it is being used by treating physicians under the routine care to treat an off-label indication which demonstrates efficacy while maintaining consistent safety profile. One of the notable examples is Ibrance (palbociclib) a kinase inhibitor indicated for the treatment of adult patients with hormone receptor (HR)-positive, human epidermal growth factor receptor 2 (HER2)-negative advanced or metastatic breast cancer in combination with another agent.

It was first approved based on a randomized trial in females. Subsequently, the approval was expanded to males and was based on real-world data from electronic health records and post-marketing records of the use of Ibrance in male patients: "Based on limited data from post-marketing reports and electronic health records, the safety profile for men treated with Ibrance is consistent with the safety profile in women treated with Ibrance."[30]

In July 2021, FDA approved Prograf (tacrolimus) for use in combination with other immunosuppressant drugs to prevent organ rejection in adult and pediatric patients receiving lung transplantation based on a non-interventional (observational) study providing RWE of effectiveness.[31] Prograf was originally approved to prevent organ rejection in patients receiving liver transplants and thereafter was approved to prevent organ rejection for kidney and heart transplants as well. However, the drug has also been routinely used in clinical practice for patients receiving lung transplants. The Sponsor used the data from the U.S. Scientific Registry of Transplant Recipients (SRTR), supported by the Department of Health and Human Services. Confirmatory evidence of effectiveness was a consequence of the RWE from the non-interventional study and randomized controlled trials of Prograf use in other solid organ transplant settings. "This approval reflects how a well-designed, non-interventional study relying on fit-for-purpose real-world data (RWD), when compared with a suitable control, can be considered adequate and well-controlled under FDA regulations."[32]

5.7 Conclusion

In summary, RWE has many uses in support of rare diseases during the drug development cycle. Application of each use needs to be considered in the context of the research question followed by a corresponding due diligence and fit-for-purpose assessment. RWE provides to the totality of evidence with respect to our understanding of the disease and/or therapy under assessment.

References

1. Cave A, Kurz X, Arlett P. Real-world data for regulatory decision making: challenges and possible solutions for Europe. *Clin Pharmacol Ther*. 2019 Jul;106(1):36–39.
2. US Food and Drug Administration. Framework for FDA's real world evidence program. Updated December 2018. Available at https://www.fda.gov/media/120060/download. Last accessed November 23, 2021.

3. ISPE's position on Real World Evidence (RWE). Available at https://pharmaco-epi.org/pub/?id=136DECF1-C559-BA4F-92C4-CF6E3ED16BB6#:~:text=ISPE%20 encourages%20the%20use%20of, medicines%20and%20other%20health%20 interventions. Last accessed November 23, 2021.
4. Flynn R, Plueschke K, Quinten C, Strassmann V, Duijnhoven RG, Gordillo-Marañon M, Rueckbeil M, Cohet C, Kurz X. Marketing authorization applications made to the European Medicines Agency in 2018–2019: what was the contribution of real-world evidence? *Clin Pharmacol Ther.* 2022 Jan;111(1):90–97.
5. Ball R, Robb M, Anderson S, Dal Pan G. The FDA's sentinel initiative—a comprehensive approach to medical product surveillance. *Clin Pharmacol Ther.* 2016;99:265–268.
6. Platt, R, Brown JS, Robb M, McClellan M, Ball R, Nguyen MD, Sherman RE. The FDA sentinel initiative—an evolving national resource. *N Engl J Med.* 2018;379:2091–2093.
7. United States Department of Health and Human Services. Food and Drug Administration. Center for Drug Evaluation and Research (CDER), Center for Biologics Evaluation and Research (CBER), and Oncology Center of Excellence (OCE). *Draft Guidance for Industry: Rare Diseases: Natural History Studies for Drug Development.* Rockville, MD: US FDA. March 2019.
8. ENCePP. Guide on Methodological Standards in Pharmacoepidemiology. Available at https://www.encepp.eu/standards_and_guidances/methodologi-calGuide.shtml. Last accessed November 23, 2021.
9. United States Department of Health and Human Services. Food and Drug Administration. Center for Drug Evaluation and Research (CDER), Center for Biologics Evaluation and Research (CBER), and Oncology Center of Excellence (OCE). *Draft Guidance for Industry: Real-World Data: Assessing Electronic Health Records and Medical Claims Data to Support Regulatory Decision-Making for Drug and Biological Products.* Rockville, MD: US FDA. September 2021.
10. Orsini, LS, Berger ML, Crown W, Daniel G, Eichler HG, Goettsch W, Graff J, Guerino J, Jonsson P, Lederer NM, Monz B. Improving transparency to build trust in real-world secondary data studies for hypothesis testing—why, what, and how: recommendations and a road map from the Real-World Evidence Transparency Initiative. *Value Health.* 2020;23(9):1128–1136.
11. European Medicines Agency. Committee for Human Medicinal Products (CHMP). *Guideline on Registry-Based Studies.* Amsterdam: EMA. 16 September 2021.
12. FDA Real-World Data: Assessing Registries to Support Regulatory Decision-Making for Drug and Biological Products Guidance for Industry. Available at https://www.fda.gov/regulatory-information/search-fda-guidance-doc-uments/real-world-data-assessing-registries-support-regulatory-decision-making-drug-and-biological-products
13. European Medicines Agency. Committee for Human Medicinal Products (CHMP). *Patient Registry Initiative- Strategy and Mandate of the Cross-Committee Task Force.* EMA Initiative. London: 5 May 2017.
14. United States Department of Health and Human Services. Food and Drug Administration. Center for Drug Evaluation and Research (CDER), Center for Biologics Evaluation and Research (CBER), and Oncology Center of Excellence

(OCE). *Draft Guidance for Industry: Real-World Data: Assessing Registries to Support Regulatory Decision-Making for Drug and Biological Products.* Rockville, MD: US FDA. November 2021.

15. Patient Registries. Available at https://www.ema.europa.eu/en/human-regu-latory/post-authorisation/patient-registries. Last accessed November 23, 2021.
16. http://www.encepp.eu/encepp/resourcesDatabase.jsp
17. United States Department of Health and Human Services. Food and Drug Administration. Center for Drug Evaluation and Research (CDER), Center for Biologics Evaluation and Research (CBER), and Center for Devices and Radiological Health (CDRH). *Draft Guidance for Industry: FDA Use of Electronic Health Record Data in Clinical Investigations Guidance for Industry.* Rockville, MD: US FDA. July 2018.
18. Fung KW, Richesson R, Bodenreider O. Coverage of rare disease names in standard terminologies and implications for patients, providers, and research. In *AMIA Annual Symposium Proceedings 2014* (Vol. 2014, p. 564). American Medical Informatics Association. 2014.
19. Garcelon N, Burgun A, Salomon R, Neuraz A. Electronic health records for the diagnosis of rare diseases. *Kidney Int.* 2020 Apr;97(4):676–686.
20. Gini R, Sturkenboom MCJ, Sultana J, Cave A, Landi A, Pacurariu A, Roberto G, Schink T, Candore G, Slattery J, Trifirò G; Working Group 3 of ENCePP (Inventory of EU Data Sources and Methodological Approaches for Multisource Studies). Different strategies to execute multi-database studies for medicines surveillance in real-world setting: a reflection on the European model. *Clin Pharmacol Ther.* 2020 Aug;108(2):228–235.
21. Manack A, Turkel CC, Kaplowitz H. (2012). Role of epidemiological data within the drug development lifecycle: a chronic migraine case study. In *Epidemiology-Current Perspectives on Research and Practice*, edited by Nuno Lunet. Rijeka, Crotia: InTech. 2012 Mar 13.
22. Leadley RM, Lang S, Misso, K, Bekkering T, Ross J, Akiyama T, Fietz M, Giugliani R, Hendriksz CJ, Hock NL, McGill J. A systematic review of the prevalence of Morquio A syndrome: challenges for study reporting in rare diseases. *Orphanet J Rare Dis.* 2014;9:173.
23. United States Department of Health and Human Services. Food and Drug Administration. Drug development for very rare diseases. Available at https://www.fda.gov/industry/orphan-products-development-events/drug-develop-ment-very-rare-diseases. Last accessed November 23, 2021.
24. Strengthening the reporting of observational studies in epidemiology. Available at https://www.strobe-statement.org/. Last accessed November 23, 2021.
25. Mistry PK, Belmatoug N, vom Dahl S, Giugliani R. Understanding the natural history of Gaucher disease. *Am J Hematol.* 2015 Jul;90(Suppl 1):S6–11.
26. ICH Harmonized Guideline: Choice of Control Group and Related Issues in Clinical Trials E10.2000. FDA Guidance. E10 Choice of Control Group and Related Issues in clinical Trials. 2001.
27. Thorlund K, Dron L, Park JJH, Mills EJ. Synthetic and external controls in clinical trials - a primer for researchers. *Clin Epidemiol.* 2020;12:457–467. doi:10.2147/CLEP.S242097

28. Seeger JD, Davis KJ, Iannacone MR, Zhou W, Dreyer N, Winterstein AG, Santanello N, Gertz B, Berlin JA. Methods for external control groups for single arm trials or long-term uncontrolled extensions to randomized clinical trials. *Pharmacoepidemiol Drug Saf.* 2020 Nov;29(11):1382–1392.
29. Burcu M, Dreyer NA, Franklin JM, Blum MD, Critchlow CW, Perfetto EM, Zhou W. Real-world evidence to support regulatory decision-making for medicines: Considerations for external control arms. *Pharmacoepidemiol Drug Saf.* 2020 Oct;29(10):1228–1235.
30. https://www.accessdata.fda.gov/drugsatfda_docs/label/ 2019/207103s008lbl.pdf
31. https://www.fda.gov/drugs/news-events-human-drugs/fda-approves-new-use-transplant-drug-based-real-world-evidence
32. https://www.fda.gov/drugs/news-events-human-drugs/fda-approves-new-use-transplant-drug-based-real-world-evidence

6

Clinical Development of Pediatric Program within Rare Diseases

Jingjing Ye
BeiGene

Lian Ma, Amy Barone, Nicholas Richardson,
Emily Wearne, Kerry Jo Lee, and Charu Gandotra
US Food and Drug Administration (FDA)

Disclaimer: This chapter reflects the views of the authors and should not be construed to represent FDA's views or policies. KJ Lee contributed Section 6.1.3, C. Gondotra contributed Section 6.1.1.

CONTENTS

DOI: 10.1201/9781003080954-6

6.1 Motivating Examples and Background

6.1.1 Motivating Examples

According to National Institutes of Health (NIH), there are approximately 7,000 rare diseases affecting between 25 and 30 million Americans. Among those, approximately 50% of the people affected by rare diseases are children. Children can benefit tremendously from new therapies, especially when the rare diseases are due to genetic deficiency, to live a longer life with quality.

In the USA, drugs being developed for children are subject to the same evidentiary standards for efficacy and safety as drugs developed in adults (see 21CFR 314.50 and PHS Act, 505(d)), that is, effectiveness is determined based on adequate and well-controlled investigations. This is also echoed by the European Medicines Agency (EMA) where marketing authorization (MA) is granted based on the provision of adequate evidence on clinical efficacy and safety.

Children as a vulnerable population in clinical research require special considerations to minimize the risk and assure prospect of direct clinical benefit when the risk to the child is more than minimal (Bavdekar, 2013). To find balance between protecting children against unknown risks and harms which may occur with trial participation and the obligation to conduct trials, children should not be enrolled in studies that are duplicative or unlikely to yield important knowledge applicable to children about the product or condition under investigation (Roth-Cline and Nelson, 2014). In this regard, both the US and EU regulations suggest a complementary strategy based on assessing the relevance of existing information in the adult population to the pediatric population, in terms of the disease, drug pharmacology, and clinical response to treatment in order to identify the gaps or level of uncertainty that need to be addressed to extend conclusion of adequate evidence of efficacy and safety (US Food and Drug Administration (FDA), 2014; EMA, 2018). This strategy is called "pediatric extrapolation" and is adopted broadly by ICH member parties to maximize the use of preexisting information and to reduce the amount of, or general need for, additional information to reach conclusions of effective and safe use of drugs in children. Partial-onset seizures (POSs), one type of epilepsy, are such an example.

Partial-onset seizures are in both adults and children, and the antiepileptic drugs (AEDs) used to treat them may have similar effects. With increasing knowledge on the disease and treatment in children, extrapolation of efficacy data from adult AEDs has been proposed as a predictive tool for assessing efficacy in children as an alternative to randomized, double-blind, placebo-controlled clinical trials in children. A first systematic study by Pellock et al. (2012) reviewed 30 adjunctive therapy trials of both POSs and primary generalized tonic-clonic seizures in adults and children aged 2–18 years. The review supports the extrapolation of efficacy results in adults to predict a similar adjunctive treatment response in children 2–18 years of age with POS. Following the Pellock review, the FDA conducted systematic and quantitative analyses of AEDs approved for use in pediatric patients. Data from 26 placebo-controlled trials in over 4,600 adults and 1,400 children aged 4 years and older were analyzed to compare responses and exposures at the approved doses between adults and age groups in children. In 2018, the FDA concluded the relationship between exposure and response (reduction in seizure frequency) in adults and children was sufficiently similar to allow for extrapolation from adult to pediatric patients 4 years and older (Ollivier et al., 2019). Further evidence supports the extrapolation down to children aged 2–4 years. FDA issued draft guidance to allow POS full extrapolation of efficacy from adults to pediatric patients of 2 years of age and above in 2019 (US Food and Drug Administration (FDA), 2019g).

Pediatric DCM is a serious and life-threatening condition. The incidence of DCM in a pediatric population in North America is 44 per million per year in infants younger than 1 year and 3.4 per million per year in children 1–18 years of age, and 1- and 5-year rates of death or transplantation are 31% and 46%, respectively. The etiology, pathophysiology, and symptoms of DCM, including edema, dyspnea, and exercise intolerance, generally overlap between adults and children. The only approved therapies for pediatric patients with HF due to DCM include ivabradine, to be used in patients who have an elevated heart rate, and sacubitril/valsartan (Entresto).

Entresto is a first-in-class neprilysin inhibitor/angiotensin receptor blocker, initially approved by the FDA in 2015 to reduce the risk of cardiovascular death (CV) and hospitalization for heart failure (HHF) in adult patients with chronic heart failure with reduced ejection fraction (HFrEF). It is a fixed-dose combination of sacubitril, a neprilysin inhibitor, and valsartan, an angiotensin receptor blocker. Neprilysin inhibition leads to increased level of peptides that are degraded by neprilysin, such as natriuretic peptides. The pharmacodynamic (PD) effects of sacubitril expected to be observed after a single dose of Entresto include increased levels of brain natriuretic peptide (BNP), that is metabolized by neprilysin; increased plasma and urinary levels of cyclic guanosine monophosphate, which is a downstream messenger of BNP; and possibly increased levels of N-terminal pro-brain natriuretic peptide (NT-proBNP).

Entresto's initial approval was based on the pivotal PARADIGM-HF trial that demonstrated efficacy of Entresto compared to enalapril in reducing the rate of CV death and HHF in adults with HFrEF. In addition, Entresto reduced the level of biomarker NT-proBNP, and the observed change from baseline at 1 month in NT-proBNP was shown statistically to explain >80% of the observed clinical benefit of Entresto in adults with HFrEF. Hence, NT-proBNP was accepted as a bridging biomarker to demonstrate efficacy of Entresto in a pediatric DCM population, and PANORAMA-HF trial was conducted in response to a pediatric written request. When agreeing to the use of NT-proBNP as the bridging biomarker, the hypothesis was that if the changes in NT-proBNP tracked similarly for both Entresto and enalapril to what was seen in adults, the clinical benefit on HF outcomes from adults can then be translated to pediatric patients.

PANORAMA-HF was an international, phase-3, two-part trial. Part 1 was an open-label study to determine the safety, tolerability, pharmacokinetics (PK), and PD of one or two oral doses of Entresto in 18 pediatric HF patients with systemic left-ventricular systolic dysfunction consistent with DCM (LVEF ≤45% or LV fractional shortening ≤22.5%). Eligible patients were placed into three age groups (Age Group 1: 6 years – <18 years, Age Group 2: 1 year – <6 years, and Age Group 3: 1 month – <1 year) that were enrolled sequentially from eldest to youngest age group. The PK of Entresto in Age Groups 1 and 2 was similar to that of adults. There were relatively few subjects with pre- and postdose PD data—a maximum of seven subjects. Therefore, reliable models of PK/PD relationship could not be generated.

Part 2 was a 52-week randomized, double-blind, parallel group, active controlled study to evaluate the efficacy, safety, and tolerability of Entresto compared with enalapril in pediatric patients with DCM. Part 2 also included an interim analysis of the NT-proBNP change from baseline at Week 12, adjusted for baseline NT-proBNP. The estimand was the change from baseline in log NT-proBNP to Week 12, expressed as a ratio of the geometric means of the

Week 12 value divided by the baseline value. The two treatment arms were compared using ANCOVA. Age, New York Heart Association/ROSS class group at randomization, region, and treatment group were included in the model as fixed-effect factors. Baseline log(NT-proBNP) and age-by-baseline log(NT-proBNP) interaction were included as covariates. Imputation for missing NT-proBNP values was conducted.

Only patients with NT-proBNP values at baseline were included in the analysis. For each patient, among all nonmissing NT-proBNP assessments (scheduled or unscheduled) after Week 4, the assessment closest to the target date (Week 12) was used to impute the missing assessment value at Week 12. The target date (Week 12) was defined as randomization date plus 84 days. After step 1, the missing NT-proBNP value at Week 12 was imputed using a multiple imputation approach based on the missing-at-random (MAR) assumption. The imputation model was a linear regression model specified using fully conditional specifications, in which the response variable was the log(NTproBNP) at Week 12; NYHA/ROSS class group at randomization and region were included as fixed-effect factors, and baseline log(NTproBNP) and the age-by-baseline log(NT-proBNP) interactions were included as covariates. For each age group and each arm, the imputation model was fitted separately based on the data from all patients in the corresponding treatment group within the age group. For each imputed dataset, the primary analysis ANCOVA model was fitted. The results were combined using Rubin's rules. To explore the robustness of the MAR assumption for the primary analysis, a sensitivity analysis based on pattern mixture model was performed to assess the case where the data were missing-not-at-random. For each patient, among all nonmissing NT-proBNP assessments (scheduled or unscheduled) after Week 4, the assessment closest to the target date (Week 12) was used to impute the missing assessment value at Week 12. After step 1, a multiple imputation approach based on pattern mixture models was applied (Carpenter and Kenward, 2013), whereby all missing data of patients in the Entresto arm who permanently discontinue the double-blind study treatment due to adverse events were assumed to behave like patients in the enalapril arm after the study treatment discontinuation and were imputed based on the data from patients in the enalapril arm. The imputation model was a linear regression model with log(NTproBNP) at Week 12 as response variable, NYHA/ROSS class group at baseline and region as fixed-effect factors, and baseline log(NT-proBNP) as covariate. The imputation model was fitted separately for each age group. After step 2, for each imputed dataset from step 2, the imputed values of the NTproBNP at the Week 12 were multiplied by a penalty factor (range from 1 to 2), if the patient had a Category 1 event (death, listing for heart transplant, or requiring VAD/ECMO/mechanical ventilation/intra-aortic balloon pump for life support) prior to Week 12.

Part 2 interim analysis included results from total 110 patients, 55 each in Entresto and enalapril arm. The baseline demographic and key disease-related characteristics were generally similar between the two treatment arms.

The adjusted geometric mean ratio of change from baseline to Week 12 for NT-proBNP for Entresto versus enalapril was 0.84 with a 95% confidence interval of 0.67–1.06, *p*-value of 0.15. Although the result was not statistically significant, the percent change in NT-proBNP observed in PANORAMA-HF was similar to that observed in PARADIGM-HF and was considered reasonably likely to translate into clinical benefit for patients with pediatric patients 1–<18 years of age with DCM. There was little difference in CV event rates and safety results between the two treatment arms in PANORAMA-HF, but there very few events in either arm. Given similar results for the bridging biomarker of NT-proBNP in pediatric patients with DCM and adult patients with HFrEF, Entresto was approved for treatment of HF due to systemic left-ventricular systolic dysfunction in pediatric patients of 1 year and older.

The rest of the chapter is structured as follows: Section 6.1.2 provides regulatory history and background for pediatric programs and approvals, in both FDA and the rest-of-the-world. Section 6.1.3 discusses the importance of natural history of rare diseases and the role of patient advocacy in drug development in rare diseases. Nonclinical and preclinical models that are applicable to pediatric programs in rare disease are included in Section 6.1.4. Section 6.2 describes pediatric extrapolation: when pediatric population can be extrapolated, the type of extrapolation and the sources of extrapolation. When no extrapolation or partial extrapolation is considered in the pediatric programs in rare disease, the trial design considerations are discussed in Section 6.3. Section 6.4 focuses on the role of modeling and simulation and key approaches with examples in facilitating pediatric drug development for rare disease. Bayesian approaches in pediatric program in rare disease to improve trial efficiencies, with respect to existing methods and considerations of utilizing existing data from adult/other age group and external controls, are discussed in Section 6.5. Other aspects including special formulations, data-sharing, and other discussions are included in Section 6.6.

6.1.2 Regulatory Consideration for Pediatric Program and Approvals

6.1.2.1 Background

United States (US) regulatory history is in large part, based on tragedies that occurred in children. Until the early 20th century, products used as medicine could be made by anyone and sold for any use; there were no federal laws to regulate this industry which was protected by the idea of free enterprise. Several important tragedies affecting children resulted in the establishment of the modern legal and regulatory framework for drug development. In 1901, 13 children died after receiving horse antiserum intended to protect against diphtheria; the antitoxin was unknowingly contaminated with tetanus toxin (US Food and Drug Administration (FDA), 2018b). A second incident involved nine children dying after receiving contaminated smallpox vaccine. These incidents and other media reports led to the implementation of two important laws: the

Biologics Control Act (1902) and the Pure Food and Drug Act (1906) (US Food and Drug Administration (FDA), 2018b). The Biologics Control Act of 1902 was intended to ensure safety and purity of serums, vaccines, and similar products intended for human use; it mandated that manufacturers in the USA be licensed annually for the manufacture and sale of antitoxins, serum, and vaccines. The Food and Drugs Act (FD&C) required that active ingredients be placed on the label of a drug's packaging and that drugs could not fall below purity levels; it also prohibited interstate commerce in misbranded and adulterated foods, drinks, and drugs (US Food and Drug Administration (FDA), 2018b). The FD&C was the basis for what is the modern US Food and Drug Administration (FDA). It is important to note that neither of these laws mandated that producers demonstrate that a drug or biologic was safe or effective, and they were essentially just required to accurately state what the product was.

Tragedy struck again in 1937 when at least 100 children died after receiving a preparation of sulfanilamide using diethylene glycol (DEG) as a solvent (US Food and Drug Administration (FDA), 2018b). At this time, animal testing was not required, and there were no regulations requiring premarket safety testing of new drugs. Under the regulations at the time, the only law that had been broken was that the company called the medicine an elixir which is a term used to describe a solvent containing ethanol (this product contained DEG). This incident led to the implantation of the 1938 Food, Drug and Cosmetic Act (FDC). The FDC required that a manufacturer proves a drug was safe prior to marketing and prohibited false therapeutic claims. The FDC did not mandate a manufacturer provides proof that a drug was effective.

It was not until 1962 with the passage of the Kefauver–Harris amendment that manufacturers were required to demonstrate that a drug was effective prior to marketing (US Food and Drug Administration (FDA), 2018b). The amendment was in response to more than 5,000 children being born with phocomelia (shortened upper limbs) in Germany after receiving thalidomide, a drug intended to treat nausea in pregnancy. Seventeen births of children with deformities linked to thalidomide were born in the USA.

It makes sense that throughout the 20th century, laws in the USA were enacted to protect children. By the 1990s however, it became apparent that the intent to protect children was actually preventing access to medications that could be studied in a well-controlled, scientific manner.

Before 1998, few drugs were approved specifically for treating pediatric diseases, although some dosing and safety information was provided in the labeling of several widely used agents (Akula et al., 2021). Most clinical trials were conducted in adults, and subsequently, healthcare providers treating children often relied on incomplete information about dosage, safety, or efficacy; they could extrapolate from these adult studies or use institutional experience when prescribing in children (Barone et al., 2019). Several publications in the literature highlight the widespread issue of using drugs to treat children where there is no indication in the product label (i.e., "off-label" use) (Sereni et al., 1975). One of the earliest reports of this was in the 1973 Physician's

Desk Reference, which stated that 78% of FDA-approved drugs lacked adequate pediatric labeling (Ristovska, 2020). In 1996, a review of pediatric medical and surgical practices stated that 25% of drugs used during hospital stays were either unlicensed or off-label (Turner et al., 1998). In the United Kingdom, a study of the National Ambulatory Medical Care survey between 2001 and 2005 showed that 62% of outpatient pediatric visits included off-label prescribing (Bazzano et al., 2009). Off-label use is particularly widespread in neonates where Conroy reported 90% of drugs used for neonates was off-label or unlicensed (Conroy et al., 1999). Conroy found that among children's wards in five hospitals in Sweden, UK, Germany, and Netherlands, 50% of all drugs were prescribed off-label or unlicensed (Conroy et al., 1999).

6.1.2.2 Pediatric Rule

In 1998, the Pediatric Rule was enacted, making it mandatory that products be required to include pediatric assessments if the drug is likely to be used in a "substantial number of pediatric patients" (50,000) or if it may provide a "meaningful therapeutic benefit" (Conroy et al., 2000). It required that sponsors include pediatric assessment of safety and efficacy in applications for new drug or biologic therapies or for new active ingredient, indications, dosage forms, new dosing regimens, or new route of administration, unless the requirement was waived or deferred (US Food and Drug Administration (FDA), 2005). A new pediatric formulation could also be required under the Pediatric Rule. The Pediatric Rule was invalidated in October 2002 in federal court under the argument that FDA's authority was exceeded by mandating sponsors to conduct pediatric studies (Association of Am. Physicians & Surgeons, Inc. v. FDA, 226 F. Supp. 2d 204 (D. D.C. 2002); however, the Pediatric Rule was the precursor for many subsequent regulations of pediatric studies including the Pediatric Research Equity Act (PREA). The Pediatric Rule was designed to work in conjunction with the pediatric exclusivity provisions of Section 505A of the Act (21 U.S.C. 355a), an incentive signed into law to encourage sponsors or holders of approved applications to voluntarily perform the pediatric studies described in a written request issued by FDA, in order to qualify for an additional 6 months of marketing exclusivity (Department of Health and Human Services (HHS), 1998).

Two laws passed by the US Congress, the PREA, which provides a requirement for pediatric studies, and the Best Pharmaceuticals for Children Act (BPCA), which provides an incentive of additional exclusivity for products of sponsors who voluntarily conduct requested studies in the pediatric population, were enacted in 2003 and 2002, respectively.

6.1.2.3 PREA

On December 3, 2003, PREA was signed into law to address the lack of pediatric use information in drug product labeling (US Food and Drug

Administration (FDA), 2005). PREA is based on similar principles as the Pediatric Rule, extending it to require pediatric studies to assess dosage, administration, safety, and efficacy for any new active ingredient, new indication, new dosage form, and new route of administration in relevant pediatric subpopulations, unless granted a waiver or deferral. In general, PREA applies only to those drugs and biological products developed for diseases and/or conditions that occur in both the adult and pediatric populations. Products intended for pediatric-specific indications will be subject to the requirements of PREA only if they are initially developed for a subset of the relevant pediatric population (HHS, 1998). Under PREA, drugs that have been granted orphan drug designation (where orphan diseases are defined as a disease with a prevalence of less than 200,000 in the USA) are exempt from PREA requirements (Section 526 is codified at 21 U.S.C. 360bb) (HHS, 1998). PREA requirements could also be waived if the indication does not occur in children or if the drug is unlikely to be used in children. For molecularly targeted therapies in oncology, the Research to Accelerate Cure and Equity (RACE) for Children Act enacted in 2017 (see discussion below) eliminated the exemption of PREA requirements based on orphan drug designation.

Prior to the RACE act, the requirement under PREA for pediatric evaluation of most oncology products developed for adult cancers was generally waived because the common cancers which occur in adults and which are the focus of drug discovery and development efforts are never or very rarely seen in children or because the indication or drug had been granted orphan designation (Akula et al., 2021). PREA therefore has had no impact on pediatric anticancer drug development. No drugs have been studied under PREA for pediatric oncology indications. Pediatric oncology trials for labeling updates are largely conducted through BPCA by the fulfillment of a written request (WR), issued by the FDA (discussed more below).

If a sponsor does not comply with PREA requirements, the FDA can label it as "misbranded" and can publicly post noncompliance letters for pediatric studies that have not been conducted by the specified due date. Additionally, the FDA can post PREA noncompliance letters if the sponsor has failed to seek or obtain a deferral extension, or has failed to apply for pediatric approval by a specified deadline. The FDA cannot withdraw marketing approval due to noncompliance with PREA (Barone et al., 2019).

6.1.2.4 The Research to Accelerate Cure and Equity (RACE) for Children Act

Section 504 of the FDA Reauthorization Act of 2017 (FDARA) amended Section 505B (also known as PREA) of the FD&C Act to require—for original applications submitted on or after August 18, 2020—pediatric investigations of certain targeted cancer drugs with new active ingredients, based on molecular mechanism of action rather than clinical indication (US Food and Drug Administration (FDA), 2019e). These amendments are sometimes referred to as the RACE for Children Act. As mentioned, prior to these amendments, most new drugs for the treatment of cancer were exempt from PREA assessment requirements because the drug was being developed for a cancer that rarely or never occurs in children making necessary studies impossible or highly impracticable, or because orphan drug designation had been granted. There is growing evidence to suggest however that genetic and other molecular biologic targets seen in adult cancers also exist in pediatric cancers. Many new targeted drugs being developed to treat oncology indications may be effective in the treatment of pediatric patients with cancer, even if the adult cancer implication does not occur in the pediatric population.

The amendments enacted by Congress in 2017 authorized FDA to require pediatric studies for certain new targeted cancer drugs or biologics based on the drug's molecular target rather than clinical indication (US Food and Drug Administration (FDA), 2019e). Specifically, if an original NDA or BLA is for a new active ingredient, and the drug that is the subject of the application is intended for treatment of an adult cancer and directed at a molecular target FDA determines to be substantially relevant to the growth or progression of a pediatric cancer, reports on the molecularly targeted pediatric cancer investigation required under Section 505B(a)(3) of the FD&C Act must be submitted with the marketing application, unless the required investigations are waived or deferred. This requirement for pediatric investigations applies even if the adult cancer indication does not occur in the pediatric population, and, per Section 505B(k)(2) of the FD&C Act, even if the drug is for an adult indication for which orphan designation has been granted.

Early advice meetings (Type F meetings) with sponsors to discuss pediatric development plans are provided in FDARA Section 503 (US Food and Drug Administration (FDA), 2020d). In situations where a conventionally designed pediatric trial may be inefficient or difficult to conduct given the rarity of affected pediatric patients, FDA encourages sponsors to request feedback from FDA early through a Type F meeting with the Oncology Center of Excellence Pediatric Oncology Program. In a Type F meeting, medical officers with board certification in pediatric oncology, and select members of the Oncology Subcommittee of the Pediatric Review Committee (PeRC) (although not in their official PeRC capacity) through the appropriate review division or office, may provide advice on the development of the iPSP. These meetings are intended to provide an opportunity to discuss the agency's current thinking about the relevance of a specific target and the expectations for early assessment in the pediatric population unless justification for a waiver or deferral of a pediatric study can be provided (US Food and Drug Administration (FDA), 2020d). Some examples of options to maintain the objective of early pediatric assessment and still satisfy the requirements of Section 505B of the FD&C Act include adding pediatric cohorts to existing adult trials, lowering the age of adult trolls to allow adolescent patients, tissue agnostic studies where multiple pediatric cancers may share genetic aberrations and could be studied with adult patients with the same aberrations, and utilization of master protocols.

6.1.2.5 BPCA

On January 4, 2002, the BPCA (Public Law 107-109) was enacted (US Food and Drug Administration (FDA), 2005; Food and Drug Administration Modernization Act of 1997, n.d.). BPCA is a voluntary program that allows FDA to issue written requests (WRs) to sponsors requesting studies of drugs and biologics to obtain additional information (e.g., dosage, safety, and efficacy) for the pediatric population where necessary. BPCA was made permeant in 2012 under the Food and Drug Administration and Safety and Innovation Act (FDASIA).

The FDA has generally issued a WR for the evaluation of a drug in a pediatric indication different from that for which the drug was either developed or approved. A sponsor may also ask the FDA to issue a WR by submitting a proposed pediatric study request. Compliance with the requirements outlined in a WR provides the company with a 6-month marketing exclusivity for the entire drug moiety. A study does not have to be positive in order to receive the exclusivity incentive.

As BPCA has been the only legislative initiative that impacts pediatric cancer drug development, more recent WRs were issued for products early in development to accelerate pediatric assessment, and requirements for studies included in the WRs were contingent upon the results of a preceding study.

Studies conducted as a requirement under PREA may also be used to support a WR; however, FDA will not issue a WR or grant exclusivity for studies that have been submitted to the agency before the WR is issued. In addition, it is important to note that a WR will often extend to the use of the active moiety for all indications that occur in the pediatric population, regardless of the indications that have been previously approved in adults or for those indications being sought in adults (US Food and Drug Administration (FDA), 2005).

6.1.2.6 Regulations in Europe and Key Comparisons to US Regulations

The European Union (EU) regulatory framework is based on a single legislation, the Pediatric Regulation, enacted in 2006 and effective as of 2007 (EMA, n.d.). The Pediatric Regulation is intended to encourage drug development for pediatric use and to ensure that drugs are safe and effective for pediatric use. The Pediatric Regulation requires that a Pediatric Investigation Plan (PIP) be submitted to the Pediatric committee for any new or existing product applying for a new indication, new route of administration, or new formulation. A PIP must include an outline of studies and a timeline required to complete studies in order to obtain MA by the EMA. Unlike PREA, the Pediatric Regulation is not limited by the indication of the product, but can incorporate a broader definition of a disease. Additionally, products that treat rare diseases or have orphan drug designation are not exempt from the Pediatric Regulation. Sponsors must complete studies outlined in the PIP prior to applying for MA, unless waived or deferred. Completion of required studies in the PIP can result in a 6-month extension of marketing exclusivity or a 2-year extension of marketing exclusivity if the product has orphan drug designation.

Under the Pediatric Regulation, submission of a PIP can be waived if the product is unlikely to be effective in pediatric patients, if the product may be unsafe in children, if the indication that the product treats does not occur in children, if the product does not provide a significant therapeutic benefit over existing pediatric therapy, if the pediatric studies cannot be performed (e.g., rare disease), or if clinical studies are not expected to be beneficial for pediatric patients. Off-patent drugs are automatically waived from the Pediatric Regulation, but a Pediatric-Use Marketing Authorization can be issued which grants 8 years of data protection and 2 years of marketing exclusivity for formulations developed exclusively for pediatric patients.

6.1.2.7 Global Implications and International Collaboration

Due to the rarity of many pediatric diseases, which are frequently subdivided into even rarer subpopulations based on underlying molecular features, international collaboration is increasingly important for facilitating the development of new treatments. Global coordination is increasingly important for prioritizing drugs of interest in general and for specific pediatric diseases, especially for drugs of the same class, for early pediatric evaluation. Several regulatory efforts exist that are intended to facilitate coordinated, global approaches to pediatric drug development:

- Pediatric cluster teleconferences: Informal teleconferences between the FDA and the EMA, together with representatives from Heath Canada, the Japanese Pharmaceutical and Medical Devices Agency, and the Australian Therapeutic Good Administration, are held at least monthly and are coordinated by FDA's Office of Pediatric Therapeutics (US Food and Drug Administration (FDA), 2020b).

- Common commentary process: The common commentary process was established by the FDA and the EMA to inform sponsors of the outcome of discussions from the pediatric cluster teleconferences. The process is intended to facilitate early interactions with sponsors and relevant agencies, not to alter or replace routine practices. The document is not binding and does provide final regulatory decisions (US Food and Drug Administration (FDA), 2020b).

- Parallel scientific advice (PSA): PSA provides a formal mechanism for provision of concurrent exchange of advice from EMA and FDA with sponsors on scientific issues to optimize drug development (General Principals EMA-FDA Parallel Scientific Advice (Human Medicinal Products), 2017).

For products being developed for the treatment of cancer for pediatric patients, FDA also encourages participation in the Pediatric Strategy Forums, organized by the ACCELERATE Platform. This is a multi-stakeholder forum of sponsors, investigators, patient advocates, and regulators to discuss development strategies for specific pediatric cancers in the context of available investigational drugs.

6.1.2.7.1 Inclusion of Adolescent Patients in Adult Oncology Trials

Adolescents have historically been excluded from adult trials based on their age, potentially delaying access to effective therapy. Adolescents (defined as ages 12–17 years of age) with cancers similar in histology and biologic behavior to those found in adults should be considered eligible for enrollment in adult oncology clinical trials (US Food and Drug Administration (FDA), 2019c). Some examples of diseases include central nervous system (CNS) tumors, melanoma, soft tissue and bone sarcoma, leukemia, and lymphoma. Enrollment of adolescents may depend on the stage of development. For first-in-human or for dose-escalation trials, it may be appropriate to include adolescents after some initial adult pharmacokinetic and toxicity data are obtained. For activity-estimating and confirmatory trials where there is more clinical experience with the drug, it may be appropriate to enroll adolescents simultaneously with adults.

Systemic exposure and clearance of drugs are generally similar in adolescent and adult patients, with 40 kg generally being the lower end of body weight range that has no clinically relevant effect on drug safety or pharmacokinetics (Chuk et al., 2017). Safety data, pharmacokinetic data, and PD data should be collected from adolescent patients who are enrolled on adult oncology trials; these data should be analyzed for any age-related differences. Additionally, sponsors should develop a plan for developmental toxicities that may require a longer duration of follow-up than is feasible in the context of an early-phase trial (e.g., growth plate abnormalities, fertility issues) (Leighton et al., 2016).

Unless adult clinical and/or nonclinical data do not provide sufficient information on toxicity, juvenile animal studies are not routinely needed before the enrollment of adolescent patients in adult oncology clinical trials (Leighton et al., 2016; Ristovska, 2020).

6.1.2.7.2 Pediatric Rare Disease Priority Review Voucher

The Rare Disease Priority Review Voucher program was enacted under Section 529 to the Federal Food, Drug and Cosmetic Act (FD&C Act) through the 2012 Food and Drug Administration Safety and Innovation Act (FDASIA) and was reauthorized under the Advancing Hope Act of 2016 (US Food and Drug Administration (FDA), 2019l; Barone et al., 2019). The program is intended to provide incentive for the developmental efforts needed to collect clinical data in rare pediatric populations of patients where an adult indication is not being sought. If granted, a voucher offers a sponsor priority review of any subsequent drug application; the voucher does not have to be used for a pediatric or orphan disease indication, and it can be transferable to another company (US Food and Drug Administration (FDA), 2019l).

6.1.3 Patient Advocacy and Natural History

Patient engagement is an important aspect of drug development. Patients are the most informed on what it means to live with their conditions. In pediatrics, a disease has a global effect on the entire family. Patients and their caregivers can inform drug development about the impact of disease and the ability to participate in clinical trials. Patients are the experts in multiple aspects of their disease, including how it relates to the following:

- The signs and symptoms of disease or condition.
- The burden of living with or managing a disease or condition.
- Barriers and difficulties of treatment (and the degree of unmet need).
- Barriers and burden of participating in clinical trials (particularly difficult in rare diseases) (US Food and Drug Administration (FDA), 2020c).

The FDA has a strong history of working to incorporate the patient voice into informing drug product development. The FDA is also developing a series of guidances regarding methodological considerations in the collection and use of patient experience data as described under the 21st Century Cures Act of 2016 Section 3002 (c) and the FDA Reauthorization Act of 2017 (FDARA), Title I) (US Food and Drug Administration (FDA), 2019i) and (US Food and Drug Administration (FDA), 2020c).

Patient input can be especially impactful early in drug development, before trials begin, to help outline the following considerations:

- Expectations of benefits (and what is most clinically meaningful to patients).
- Tolerance for harms or risks.
- Acceptable trade-offs of benefits and risks (i.e., patient preference).
- Attitudes toward uncertainty.

FDA routinely meets with patients to hear from them in patient-listening sessions and patient-focused drug development meetings. Information learned from patients can be used to inform clinical trial design. In rare diseases, small patient populations can limit the number of trials performed. Therefore, it is important for drug developers to involve patients early in drug development to design trials with considerations that are most meaningful to patients while generating evidence regarding the safe and effective use of therapies.

The EMA similarly routinely solicits patient input into the drug development of rare diseases. They have a framework for their interaction with patients and highlight that it aims at the following[1,2]:

- Supporting the agency to access experiences of diseases, their management, and information on current use of medicines,

- Contributing to more efficient and targeted communication to patients and consumers, and
- Enhancing understanding of the role of the EU medicines regulatory network.

At the EMA, patients contribute to multiple facets of drug development designed to solicit patient input on disease-specific information or experience, the preparation of guidelines, and as members of scientific committees.

An important record of patient experience is in the natural history of a disease or condition. A disease's natural history can be defined as the progression of a disease process in an individual over time, in the absence of treatment (CDC). Patient experience characterizes the natural history of a disease and enhances our understanding of a condition's progression, severity, and chronicity. The definition of a natural history study is a preplanned observational study intended to track the course of the disease (National Cancer Institute (NCI), n.d.). Reliable information about the collective natural history of a condition is particularly relevant in rare diseases that are often chronic, slowly progressive, and heterogeneous either in severity or in manifestation, across multiple organ systems. Data from well-designed natural history studies are critical to inform planning in rare disease drug development programs where the same information typically generated from larger multiple-phased studies for medical product development in common diseases may not be possible in small populations (US Food and Drug Administration (FDA), 2019k). Data from these studies also provide information on the disease's demographics (including in relevant subpopulations) and genetics to inform the natural trajectory of the disease.

The data collected from well-designed natural history studies inform drug development planning in several ways. It can allow for informed selection of a relevant patient population or subset due to genotypic or phenotypic heterogeneity or treatment effect of the product (i.e., treatment of a symptom). It can also help aid selection of endpoints for clinical trials either by determining the most appropriate direct measure of clinically meaningful benefit or by tracking the potential use of clinical outcome assessments or biomarkers against outcomes that measure or demonstrate direct clinical benefit. A natural history study can additionally assist in determining the length of the trial necessary to demonstrate a clinically meaningful treatment effect. In US federal regulations, it is described that there are limited occasions where historical controls (such as derived from a natural history study) may be used as a control in an adequate and well-controlled trial "to distinguish the effect of a drug from other influences, such as spontaneous change in the course of the disease, placebo effect, or biased observation" (Code of Federal Regulations (CFR), 2020). Historical control designs are usually reserved for special circumstances, such as studies of diseases with high and predictable mortality (such as certain malignancies) and studies where the effect of the drug is self-evident (e.g., drug metabolism).

Natural history studies can be either retrospective, involving a collection of evaluations that has already occurred (e.g., medical chart review), or prospective (preplanned collection). Retrospective studies have the advantage of being more quickly performed as data may be more readily available, however, may be limited by missing or erroneous data entry or coding, the change of terminology or standard of care over time, or bias pertaining to the selection of patients to be enrolled due to timing of diagnosis, severity of illness, or successful outcomes. Patients with rare diseases are particularly vulnerable to misdiagnosis or late diagnosis, and those with the most severe manifestations of a condition may be the only ones enrolled. Prospective studies can eliminate parts of selection and historical biases and have the advantage of prospectively timing assessments in line with potential drug development programs. Prospective studies can also ensure standardization of collected data but can take longer to perform. Natural history studies can be invaluable to rare disease trial design, inform patient and endpoint selection, and are most useful to drug development if they are designed with forethought to what questions they need to answer to inform future drug development.

One real-world data source to help characterize the natural history of a disease is a registry. A registry is defined as an organized system that collects clinical and other data in a standardized format for a population defined by a particular disease, condition, or exposure (Draft Guidance: Real-World Data: Assessing Registries to Support Regulatory Decision-Making for Drug and Biological Products, Guidance for Industry 2021).[3] When evaluating the usefulness of registries to inform the natural history of a condition, one should consider the elements collected are sufficient or complete for the purpose of the study, whether the patient population selected represents the population intended for study, and whether standards or aspects of care have evolved since the registry was initiated. As with any data source, the reliability of the registry data (collection process and data integrity) should be considered.

The patient's voice and the characterization of a patient's condition through natural history studies are critical components to rare disease drug development. Rare disease drug development is complex due to the challenges of trial design with small populations, incomplete or unknown information about the condition, and the degree of unmet need. These challenges can be mitigated to some degree with early planning and outreach to gather as much information as possible to construct a rigorous drug development program designed to generate scientific evidence that is both sound and interpretable.

6.1.4 Preclinical and Nonclinical Models

Preclinical testing is crucial to protect the safety of adult and pediatric patients. Prior to initiating first-in-human (FIH) clinical studies, new investigational drugs should be evaluated in appropriately designed nonclinical studies as discussed in ICH M3(R2) Guidance for Industry: Nonclinical

Safety Studies for the Conduct of Human Clinical Trials and Marketing Authorization for Pharmaceuticals and other applicable guidances (ICH, 2010a, b, (2012); US Food and Drug Administration (FDA), 2019h). The goal of nonclinical studies at this early stage in development is to identify pharmacologic properties, identify potential target organs of toxicity to inform clinical monitoring, and establish a safe initial starting dose for FIH exposure. For oncology drugs, the FIH starting dose is generally based on Good Laboratory Practice (GLP)-compliant (see 21 CFR Part 58) repeat-dose toxicology studies [i.e., 1/10 of the severely toxic dose in 10% of the animals (STD_{10}) in rodents or 1/6 of the highest non-severely toxic dose in nonrodents; ICH S9]. For biopharmaceuticals with immune agonistic properties, selection of the starting dose using a minimally anticipated biologic effect level or pharmacological effect level may be more appropriate (US Food and Drug Administration (FDA), 2020a). For non-life-threatening diseases and patients with a longer life expectancy, a more conservative starting dose approach based on the no-observed adverse effect level in animals is used as described in ICH M3(R2).

First-in-human studies for oncology drugs are usually conducted initially in adult patients. When pediatric studies are warranted based on a drug's molecular target(s), available clinical safety data in adults can be used to support clinical studies in pediatric patients with cancer. The starting dose in pediatric patients is generally based on tolerated doses in adult patients, taking into account body surface area. In order to select appropriate agents for pediatric development, preclinical pharmacology models are often used to evaluate the potential in-vitro and in-vivo activities of drugs in pediatric cancers. These include in-vitro (cell lines and three-dimensional organoids) and in-vivo [tumors transplanted from patients to mice, i.e., patient-derived xenograft (PDX)] models of pediatric cancers, high-throughput screening, and in-silico evaluation. Nonclinical pharmacology studies can also be utilized to inform initial dosing strategies when clinical investigation is initiated in pediatric patients. In addition, there are collaborative efforts to improve access to preclinical pediatric models and prioritize which agents to pursue in pediatric clinical trials (Reaman et al., 2020), including the National Cancer Institute (NCI)-funded Preclinical Pediatric Testing Consortium (PPTC), previously known as the Pediatric Preclinical Testing Program (PPTP) (Houghton et al., 2007). Through collaboration with academic and pharmaceutical partners, the PPTC screens therapeutic agents for antitumor efficacy in genomically characterized PDX models of high-risk childhood cancers. PPTC has genomically characterized 261 PDX models from 37 unique pediatric cancers (Rokita et al., 2019). In addition, the Innovative Therapies for Children with Cancer Pediatric Preclinical Proof-of-concept Platform (ITCC-P4) was initiated in Europe in 2017 to establish PDX models of pediatric high-risk malignant tumors and leukemias. As of December 2019, 150 pediatric PDX models have been established and characterized (Reaman et al., 2020). Although PDX studies can overpredict clinical activity and are associated with other inherent limitations (Kurmasheva and Houghton, 2016), they can be an important tool in selecting and prioritizing appropriate agents for pediatric cancer clinical trials.

Nonclinical safety testing to support pediatric development is discussed in ICH S9 for oncology drugs. ICH (2021) can be consulted for juvenile animal study design if warranted. ICH S11 states that additional nonclinical studies are not warranted to support pediatric development when existing clinical safety data and risk mitigation strategies are considered sufficient to support pediatric use. ICH S11 encourages the use of a weight of evidence (WoE) approach when determining whether additional nonclinical studies including juvenile animal studies (JASs) are warranted. This WoE approach incorporates clinical context, youngest intended patient age, potential effects on developing organ systems, amount/type of existing clinical and nonclinical data, selectivity/specificity of the pharmaceutical, and clinical treatment duration. Given the utility of available clinical data in adult patients, the relatively short life expectancy of pediatric patients in Phase 1 or 2 trials, and the benefit of not delaying clinical development for pediatric patients with advanced cancer and limited therapeutic options, FDA does not generally recommend conducting toxicology studies in juvenile animals to support treatment of pediatric patients with cancer (ICH 2018); (Leighton et al., 2016)). An analysis of JAS conducted by the FDA Oncology Office in 2016 concluded that JASs conducted to date have not provided useful information to support first-in-pediatric development for anticancer pharmaceuticals (Leighton et al., 2016). Further, JAS findings did not affect any aspect of first-in-pediatric trials or pediatric dose selection (Leighton et al., 2016).

There are rare occasions, however, when FDA may consider a JAS for an anticancer pharmaceutical (e.g., dinutuximab and naxitamab). Potential examples include the absence of clinical data in adult patients (i.e., the drug is being developed exclusively for pediatric patients), when development is pursued in children with a longer life expectancy, or to address a specific safety concern or question. If a JAS is warranted based on these concerns and following consultation with the relevant FDA oncology review division, ICH S11 should be consulted regarding the design of the JAS. UNITUXIN (dinutuximab) and DANYELZA (naxitamab-GQGK) are glycolipid disialoganglioside (GD2)-binding monoclonal antibodies approved for the treatment of high-risk neuroblastoma, which is largely a disease of pediatric and young adult patients. Dinutuximab is approved for pediatric patients, and naxitamab is approved for pediatric patients of 1 year of age and older and adult patients. Given the lack of chronic toxicology studies or clinical data clearly isolating the treatment effect of dinutuximab alone, the pediatric indication, the major toxicity associated with dinutuximab (i.e., neuropathic pain), and residual uncertainty regarding the potential for recovery of peripheral nerve damage, FDA requested a postmarketing requirement (PMR) to conduct a 5-month JAS in cynomolgus monkeys with dinutuximab incorporating additional peripheral nervous system, CNS, and pain endpoints to further evaluate the potential for neurotoxicity in developing brains. For naxitamab, FDA had concerns regarding the relevance of the animal model used to assess toxicity. Given the age of the intended pediatric patient population and potential effects on nerve development, FDA requested a PMR to further explore the toxicity of naxitamab in a relevant animal species using juvenile animals.

The EMA has a slightly different perspective than the FDA on JAS. The EMA position is that although JAS should not delay pediatric trials, they serve to improve the provisions to safeguard against intolerable harm and monitor for age-specific risks (US Food and Drug Administration (FDA) & EMA, 2021). EMA encourages sponsors to reflect on the necessity of whether and by when juvenile animal data should be available. From an EMA perspective, JASs are more likely to be warranted: (1) to investigate concerns for effects on vital organs in patients below 1–2 years old with immature clearance pathways; (2) prior to initiating studies in pediatric patients with a good chance for long-term survival; (3) when there is target expression in the CNS and brain penetration; (4) when there is potential concern for toxicities that are difficult to monitor clinically or for which clinical data in adults are of limited relevance; and (5) for novel anticancer medicines targeting cell biology or developmental pathways with pleiotropic effects (EMA/FDA, 2021).

In addition to available clinical safety data in adult patients, mechanism of action (e.g., VEGFR/FGFR, TRKA/B/C inhibitors) and data from general toxicology studies in adult animals can provide insights into toxicities that may preferentially affect pediatric patients compared to adults. For example, findings in adult animals that may predict adverse effects on pediatric patient growth or development include growth plate findings (e.g., histologic physeal dysplasia), bone/teeth toxicity, and CNS findings suggestive of impaired cognitive development. Such animal findings may warrant additional monitoring in pediatric clinical studies. In addition, investigators should pay special attention to pharmaceuticals whose targets are involved in growth and organ development.

Ultimately, mechanism of action and pharmacologic models of pediatric cancers can be used to evaluate therapeutic agents preclinically prior to clinical studies in pediatric populations. Existing safety data in adult patients are often sufficient to support clinical studies in pediatric patients, along with extrapolation of developmentally relevant findings from toxicology studies conducted in adult animals.

6.2 Pediatric Extrapolation

The goal of extrapolation is to leverage existing data from a studied patient population to support a demonstration of effectiveness and, in some cases, safety in the indicated patient population. The process of extrapolation, when based on sound scientific principles, can substantially facilitate the availability of information to ultimately support safe and effective therapies for pediatric patients or patients with rare diseases. This approach can provide robust scientific evidence and encourage development programs for pediatric patients and/or patients with rare diseases. Leveraging existing clinical data to support a specific population ultimately benefits patients. For example, with clinical development of antivirals for human immunodeficiency virus (HIV) infection, the European Union guideline, in 2007, supported use of extrapolation of efficacy from adult to pediatric populations. The impact of the use of extrapolation was assessed for antiviral therapies authorized before and after 2007 for pediatric patients with HIV, which demonstrated that before 2007, 48 clinical trials (4,971 pediatric patients) were conducted to support 11 pediatric antiviral authorizations, and after 2007, 12 clinical trials (621 pediatric patients) were conducted to support 13 pediatric antiviral authorizations (Ollivier et al., 2019).

The objectives of this section are to provide practical recommendations on the considerations for when extrapolation is appropriate and the extent the existing data can be leveraged. For this section, the definition of extrapolation is to leverage existing data from a studied patient population in support of effective and safe use of drugs in the pediatric population when it can be assumed that the course of the disease and the expected response to a medicine product would be sufficiently similar in the pediatric and source (adult or other pediatric) population (US Food and Drug Administration (FDA), 2018a). The studied patient population is hereafter referred to as the *source* population to support for the pediatric or a subgroup of the pediatric or rare disease population, referred to as the *target* population.

For extrapolation, the types of clinical data to be considered include, but are not limited to, randomized controlled trials, single-arm trials, historical clinical data, published literature, and pharmacokinetic or PD data. To support a demonstration of effectiveness or safety in the indicated population, the existing clinical data can be fully or partially extrapolated (US Food and Drug Administration (FDA), 2014). For full extrapolation, the existing clinical data are intended to be used as a substitute for efficacy or safety, and no prospective clinical data in the target population are anticipated. The relevance and the quality of the data are critical attributes to determine whether full extrapolation is warranted. Notably, based on differences between adults or a separate subpopulation, full extrapolation of safety is exceedingly rare. For partial extrapolation, the existing clinical data are intended to supplement prospective clinical data in the indicated population. The use of partial extrapolation is dependent on the relevance of the extrapolated data to provide the ability to make inferences in the indicated population. Furthermore, efficacy or safety or both may be considered for extrapolation, although each should be considered separately. For instance, it may be scientifically appropriate to fully extrapolate efficacy for the indicated population, but no extrapolation or partial extrapolation for safety.

The determination of whether an extrapolation approach is appropriate is primarily based on the similarities of the existing data in source population to the target population in terms of patient characteristics, disease course, similar treatment response, and the quality of data. If the patient populations are comparable or relevant and the data quality is adequate, the prospect of extrapolation for efficacy or safety is much greater.

To determine whether extrapolation should be considered, a set of questions can be considered to determine the relevance of the existing data to the target population and the comparability of the existing data.

First, the relevance of the existing data should be assessed. For instance, for pediatric development, does the disease of interest occur in the pediatric population? Is there similarity between source and target populations based on physiology and maturation in etiology, pathophysiology, manifestation, and progression? Is the underlying pathophysiology similar between the existing clinical data and the indicated population? For example, chronic myeloid leukemia (CML) occurs primarily in adults but does occur in the pediatric population to a limited degree. Both adult and pediatric patients with CML have a similar underlying biologic driver, a BCR-ABL fusion gene.

Second, an assessment of the endpoints measured in the existing clinical data in source population and their relevance to the target population should be evaluated. Is the same or an adequately relevant endpoint measured in the existing data (i.e., adult data) as would be in the target population? For example, in adult patients with CML, a major molecular response (MMR) based on BCR-ABL expression is used to evaluate response to targeted BCR-ABL kinase inhibitor treatment in these patients. The same endpoint is used to evaluate response in pediatric patients with CML treated with the same therapies. Thus, the adult data evaluating MMR can be considered relevant to pediatric patients with CML and are appropriate to consider for extrapolation of efficacy. The initial assessment of relevance of the existing data is critical to inform whether an extrapolation approach should be further considered.

Following the assessment of relevance to the target population, the existing data should be evaluated for comparability, that is, differences between the existing data and the target population in terms of population or disease characteristics, treatment (including pharmacology on exposure and exposure–response), treatment response, or other parameters that could impact safety or effectiveness.

For population and disease characteristics, are there identified characteristics that are unique or different that may impact safety or efficacy in the target population. For example, in patients with Gaucher disease, disease-modifying factors such as mutation types, residual enzyme activity, age, and epigenetic factors result in presentations of the disease that differ between adult and pediatric patients. Further, the prevalence, severity of a disease, and the natural history of the disease may be different between adult and pediatric patients. An important aspect specific to pediatric populations is growth and development and organ maturation. If notable differences are identified that may impact safety or efficacy, full extrapolation is probably not feasible; however, partial extrapolation may still be considered once the characteristics are taken into consideration.

For treatment, differences that may impact safety or efficacy are dose, exposure, pharmacokinetics, PDs, and treatment intent. Dosing characteristics include differences in formulation (tablet or capsule versus liquid), flat dose versus weight-based dosing, differences in pharmacokinetic parameters, and treatment exposure (fixed duration versus continuous therapy). In addition, treatment may be administered as a single agent versus in combination depending on the treatment intent and the standard of care in the respective populations, all of which should be considered when evaluating whether the existing data are comparable to the indicated population. Further, the intent of treatment may be different between the existing data and the indicated population, such as treatment intended for curative intent, palliative, or supportive care. Again, if notable differences are identified, full extrapolation is likely not feasible, yet partial extrapolation can still be considered.

In evaluating treatment response, the initial evaluation of relevance of the existing data to determine whether the endpoints used in the existing data are the same or adequately similar to the target population is useful. Beyond the initial evaluation, any differences in response to treatment, in terms of safety or efficacy, should be considered. In particular, is there a rationale for the mechanism of action and thus treatment response to be different within the existing clinical data and the target population? Are there specific considerations when evaluating response to treatment?

Finally, based on the existing clinical data and the target population, are there other differences that could impact safety or efficacy? For the specific population of interest and the relevant clinical data, there may be differences that are not addressed by evaluating, the comparability of population or disease characteristics, treatment, treatment response, or pharmacokinetics. Nevertheless, if notable differences are identified, full extrapolation is likely not feasible, yet partial extrapolation can be considered depending on the identified differences and the potential impact on safety and efficacy. If there are no notable differences and the quality of the existing data is adequate, full extrapolation can be considered.

An example in which an extrapolation approach was utilized was for avelumab for the treatment of pediatric patients of 12 years and older with metastatic Merkel cell carcinoma (MCC). MCC is a rare, aggressive neuroendocrine carcinoma of the skin that is considered incurable. The mean age at presentation is 75 years, and risk factors include ultraviolet radiation, infection with Merkel cell polyomavirus, advanced age, and immunosuppression. The 5-year survival rate for patients with metastatic MCC is 25%. Prior to avelumab, there were no approved therapies for patients with metastatic MCC.

Avelumab is a monoclonal antibody against the programmed death ligand 1 (PD-L1), a PD-L1 immune-checkpoint inhibitor. The approval of avelumab was supported by the JAVELIN Merkel 200 trial (NCT02155647), which was a multicenter, single-arm trial in 88 adult patients with metastatic MCC. In 88 patients, avelumab demonstrated a clinically meaningful response rate of 33% with durability and a tolerable safety profile. To support an extrapolation approach for pediatric patients of 12 years and older, it was noted:

- There are no differences in histopathologic and virologic aspects of the disease between adult and pediatric patients.

- There is an association with the Merkel cell polyomavirus that occurs in 80% of adult patients and 60% of patients between the ages of 10 and 20 years, indicating a similar association between adults and pediatrics.

- Population pharmacokinetic (PK) modeling included simulation of PK exposure at steady state after repeat avelumab dosing for patients with body weights of 30–90 kg, which is equivalent to weights of adolescents. The results of this analysis demonstrated comparable PK between patients with body weights of 30–90 kg and adults. Also, no differences in PK based on age were observed.

- The population PK modeling simulated target occupancy, predicting high target occupancy for pediatric patients of 12 years and older with the prescribed dose and throughout the dose regimen.

- Clinical data in the published literature and from clinical trials provided some supportive information on the diagnosis, disease characteristics, and treatment for pediatric patients with MCC, supporting that treatment with avelumab in pediatrics is similar to adults.

Therefore, it was scientifically justified to use extrapolation to support a determination of effectiveness and safety for avelumab in pediatric patients of 12 years and older with metastatic Merkel cell carcinoma.

The quality of the existing clinical data plays an important role on the ability to use an extrapolation approach, full or partial extrapolation. Data quality considers the source of the data, the study design, data collection, and the applicability of the data to the indicated population. For instance, data from a randomized trial are higher quality than a single-arm trial or a patient registry. Additionally, based on the source and study design, the collection of data may be variable and may introduce bias. Moreover, the data should be applicable to the target population in respect to the disease setting and the current treatment paradigm. The confidence in the data quality is integral to the ability to borrow from the existing clinical data to support a demonstration of effectiveness or safety.

For full extrapolation, the relevance and the quality of data are critical, given that the extrapolated data will provide the clinical data to support the substantial evidence of effectiveness or safety for the target population. If there are no expected differences between the existing data in source and the target population that would impact safety or efficacy and the existing data quality is adequate, full extrapolation can be considered.

When considering use of partial extrapolation, it will be dependent on the prospective clinical data to be obtained in the target population and whether an appropriate statistical model can be incorporated to provide reliable inference by borrowing from the existing data. The model can potentially account for some of the identified differences based on the considerations described above. Therefore, the extrapolated data can be supportive, along with the prospective clinical data, to provide substantial evidence of effectiveness or safety for the treatment in the target population. Importantly, the evaluation of relevance and comparability of the existing data is conducted after the data become available and then the extent of partial extrapolation can be determined, although, if the existing data are determined to be inadequate or unreliable to support efficacy or safety, an extrapolation approach should not be considered. When extrapolation is not appropriate, adequate and well-controlled studies are necessary to provide evidence for effectiveness and safety.

The use of an extrapolation approach may be limited by a number of factors. Some considerations that preclude the use of an extrapolation approach include the following:

- Limited knowledge of the disease in the indicated population.
- The treatment is not approved in adults or a separate, relevant subpopulation.
- Endpoints are not similar.
- A valid statistical approach to account for differences is not feasible.
- Population-specific issues—pediatric growth and development.
- Differences in the natural history of the disease or the standard of care.
- Unable to provide appropriate risk mitigation.

Considerations that may limit extrapolation to a partial extrapolation approach include the following:

- Population differences—age, biomarker expression.
- Existing clinical data are not adequately representative of current treatment.
- Based on identified differences, there is uncertainty regarding the adequacy of borrowing the data to support the overall evidence of effectiveness or safety.

Ultimately, the ability to use an extrapolation approach is dependent on how any differences and the quality of the data impact the ability to borrow the existing data. Use of extrapolation, full or partial, can leverage existing data to support the overall assessment of efficacy or safety; however, extrapolation does introduce residual uncertainty. The statistical approach utilized can help address some of the uncertainty, yet the level of uncertainty is based on the differences between the existing data and the target population and should be considered to determine whether extrapolation is supportive or introduces unacceptable uncertainty, making the data uninformative. Therefore, an extrapolation approach should be based on reasonable, sound scientific considerations that allow for support of the effectiveness or safety of a treatment for the indicated population.

6.3 Trial Design Considerations When No Extrapolation or Partial Extrapolation are Used in Efficacy Add Evaluation

Statutory standards for approval of orphan drugs developed for treatment of rare diseases are the same as those of common diseases: There must be substantial safety and efficacy evidence. Adequate and well-controlled trials remain the "gold standard" to generate the substantial evidence, for pediatric disease that is dissimilar in adults or if there are no adults with disease, where extrapolation is not feasible. However, in cases when it is not possible to meet these standards, the regulators are open to discuss the adoption of alternative strategies in trial design and apply regulatory flexibility in decision-making about drug development and approval in rare diseases. The objective of this section is to provide the alternative strategies that have shown success in practice to support approvals in pediatric program within rare disease.

Drug developers may consider different design options and discuss their applicability with respect to efficiency and risk of bias. In a paper outlining the recommendations from the Small Population Clinical Trials (SPCT) Task Force of the International Rare Diseases Research Consortium (IRDiRC) (S Day et al., *Orphanet Journal of Rare Diseases*, 2019), a few alternative study design options were discussed along with the benefit and risk of each approach.

- Crossover designs: They can be considered for stable diseases with relatively short treatment duration, as they may allow potential large reductions in required sample size. Such designs allow each subject to receive both (or more than two) interventions but will not be applicable in highly variable conditions or that where very long follow-up is needed.
- Adaptive seamless designs: They may improve trial efficiency by combining an exploratory "phase 2 part" of a trial (e.g., dose-finding) with the confirmatory "phase 3 part" of the same trial. The challenges for

these designs include the time required for the design and appropriate analyses.

- Study design options that allow subjects to be used more than once (e.g., multiple n-of-1 trials, crossover trial designs, or randomized withdrawal designs).

The 2019 FDA "Draft Guidance of industry: Rare Diseases: Common Issues in Drug Development" (US Food and Drug Administration (FDA), 2019j) also suggests that the sponsors can address patient and family concerns by using modified trial designs, when appropriate, to demonstrate effectiveness and interpretation of safety signals. These alternative designs retain the advantages of placebo-controlled trials and include features that minimize placebo exposure and enhance access to experimental therapies (e.g., dose-response, delayed start, randomized withdrawal, crossover, adaptive designs with interim analysis).

6.3.1 Adaptive Design

Both FDA and EMA published guidance to provide recommendations to sponsors for the development of adaptive clinical trials (US Food and Drug Administration (FDA), 2019b; EMA, 2007). While being cautious about the risks associated with adaptive clinical trials, the document provides guidance on modifications that can be planned in a prospectively written protocol, including eligibility criteria, randomization procedure, total sample size, and endpoints. Caution should however be taken concerning the generalizability and applicability of adaptive clinical trial results. Various strategies may aim to decrease heterogeneity, improve disease characterization, and predict clinical course, which could thereby shape patient selection prior to randomization but do not generally reduce statistical validity regarding the study population. FDA and EMA furthermore encourage early communication to assist in drug evaluation, scientific and medical questions that may arise throughout the clinical investigation.

6.3.2 Multi-arm Designs/Master Protocol

Master protocols, including platform trials, basket trials, and umbrella trials, are trials that incorporate several treatments in several treatment arms, each being tested for similar (although not necessarily identical) indications, possibly sharing a common control. The different treatments and trial arms might or might not start at the same time, and treatment arms might be added or dropped as the trial progresses (Woodcock and LaVange, 2017). Larotrectinib was approved in 2018 based on a basket trial design in both pediatric and adult patients who were diagnosed with solid tumors that have a neurotrophic receptor tyrosine kinase (NTRK) gene fusion without a known acquired resistance mutation, that are either metastatic or where surgical resection likely to result in severe morbidity and who have no satisfactory alternative treatments or whose cancer has progressed following treatment ((FDA), Larotrectinib, US Prescriber Information (USPI), 2018).

Potential advantages of these types of trial designs include the following: (1) improve efficiency by sharing resources and diminish trial costs; (2) reduce patients' exposure to a placebo, thereby encouraging participation; and (3) enable comparison of active substances. There are certain challenges with these designs as follows:

- In case trial treatments are from different sponsors, there is the need for sponsors to cooperate and agree to a common protocol.
- Need for additional time to design such a complex study.
- Challenges of trial leadership and operating the clinical trial.
- Differences of interest between competitive companies, charities, and investigators.
- Potential heterogeneity and thus loss in efficiency due to heterogeneous settings.

6.3.3 Historical Control

When concurrent controls are impractical or unethical, clinical trials can rely on an external historical control. As there is no randomization to a concurrent comparator group (e.g., placebo/standard of care), the inability to eliminate systematic differences between nonconcurrent treatment groups could be a major concern. This situation generally restricts use of historical control designs to assessment of serious disease when (1) there is an unmet medical need, (2) there is a well-documented, highly predictable disease course that can be objectively measured and verified, such as high and temporally predictable mortality, and (3) there is an expected drug effect that is large, self-evident, and temporally closely associated with the intervention. A recent review paper by Lim et al. (2018) indicated that regulators in both FDA and EMA have demonstrated willingness to accept the use of historical controls when the study subjects are scarce in pediatric and rare diseases.

Natural history study providing systematically and comprehensively captured data using uniform medical language and methodologies relevant to the interventional clinical trials would help to ensure that the historical control is comparable to the treatment group. Further, for diseases with substantial heterogeneity in clinical presentation, improved predictive ability based on the natural history of the disease may inform inclusion/exclusion criteria to facilitate an effective clinical trial program and help identify potential biomarkers to guide treatment. In particular, natural history data can inform endpoint selection in the context of event rate and variability of disease presentation to ensure that the number of patients enrolled should allow sufficient power to detect efficacy.

6.3.4 Enrichment Strategies

The small sample sizes associated with studies of rare diseases can restrict study design options, replication, and the use of inferential statistics, which calls for innovative methods to assist in assessing the evidence of the efficacy and safety of a potential treatment. Enrichment is one option, wherein patients are enrolled on the basis of a prospectively defined characteristic that is believed to improve the probability of detecting a treatment effect compared with an unselected patient population. This can include defining a narrow patient population to reduce patient variability, selecting patients who have a higher probability of experiencing an endpoint, or selecting patients who are expected to be more likely to respond to treatment.

Three categories of enrichment strategies are discussed in detail in the 2019 FDA "Guidance for Industry: Enrichment Strategies for Clinical Trials to Support Determination of Effectiveness of Human Drugs and Biological Products": (1) practical enrichment, which reduces non-drug-related variability; (2) prognostic enrichment, which increases the incidence of clinical events of interest; and (3) predictive enrichment, which selects patients most likely to response to treatment (US Food and Drug Administration (FDA), 2019d).

For pediatric clinical trials, Green et al. (2018) analyzed 112 pediatric efficacy studies with 76 drug development programs submitted to the US Food and Drug Administration (US FDA) between 2012 and 2016. They reported that 88 trials employed at least one enrichment strategy in pediatric trials. In addition, the highest success rates were achieved when all three enrichment strategies (practical, predictive, and prognostic) were used together within a single trial, while the lowest success rate was observed when no enrichment strategy was used.

6.3.5 Efficacy Endpoints

Endpoint selections for a clinical trial are typically based on the following:

- The range and course of clinical manifestations associated with the disease, which can be obtained from a natural history study of the disease.
- The clinical characteristics of the specific target population, which may be a subset of the total population with a disease.
- The aspects of the disease that are meaningful to the patient and that could be assessed to evaluate the drug's effectiveness.

For many rare diseases where well-characterized efficacy endpoints are not available, establishing a biomarker or surrogate endpoint that predicts clinical benefit would be important to support the possibility of using the accelerated approval pathway.

Different endpoints are often appropriate for the evolving objectives of clinical trials. Although the earliest clinical investigations will usually focus on safety assessments, early investigations also can be useful in evaluating a drug's PK and PD effects. Sponsors should conduct early- and mid-phase (e.g., phase 2) clinical investigations to guide selection of dose regimen and can rely on PD or intermediate clinical effects, which may be seen earlier than more definitive endpoints. Late-phase clinical investigations are generally designed to provide clear determinations of efficacy and further evaluation of safety.

6.3.6 Dose Selection

When the disease pathobiology and the mechanism of action for drug would not differ by age, a starting dose may be selected by targeting similar exposure to the adult therapeutic dose without the need to evaluate multiple dose levels (full extrapolation). When similarity in disease between pediatric and adults cannot be assumed, a more extensive PK and dose-finding study in pediatric patients may be required. Examples include inborn errors of metabolism or infantile forms of disease that are fatal in childhood. Depending on the disease, the PK and safety data from healthy adults or adult patients may help inform the pediatric starting dose. When no adult data are available or testing in adults will not be informative, the starting dose may be derived from nonclinical animal models or other mechanistic in-vivo or in-vitro data, particularly if the therapy is targeted.

6.4 Application of Modeling and Simulations in the Pediatric Drug Development for Rare Disease

Model-informed drug development (MIDD) refers to the application of a wide range of quantitative models in facilitating drug development and informing decision-making. The evolution and use of MIDD in streamlining the overall drug discovery, development, and regulatory evaluation has been well documented (Lesko, 2021; Wang et al., 2019; Zhu et al., 2019; Madabushi et al., 2019). Advancing MIDD was formally recognized by FDA as one of the key performance goals and procedures in the Prescription Drug User Fee Act (PDUFA) re-authorization fiscal years 2018–2022 (PDUFA VI) (US Food and Drug Administration (FDA), n.d.-b).

Due to the nature of the disease and scarcity of patient population, there is often limited opportunity to get things right in pediatric rare disease drug development space, and thus, maximizing the use of all available data is in the interest for the drug developers and regulators. This brings opportunities for MIDD approaches to utilize and integrate all available sources and knowledge to quantitatively assess benefit/risk and dosing decisions. As described previously by Bi et al, the MIDD applications in pediatric drug development can be broadly classified into three categories: (1) leveraging knowledge for bridging the gap, (2) supporting dose selection and optimization, and (3) informing clinical trial design (Bi et al., 2019). Similar applications have been employed for pediatric drug development in rare disease to improve efficiency and success rate of the trials.

6.4.1 Dose Selection and Extrapolation

Data from the adult disease programs may provide support evidence for efficacy and extrapolation. Such data could be used in exploring differences in pharmacokinetic (PK), PK/PDs (PD), and clinical response to treatment in the pediatric population. Model-based approaches, such as population PK (popPK) models and physiologically based pharmacokinetic (PBPK) models, are commonly used to derive pediatric dosing regimens with the goal of matching the safe and effective exposure that was established in adult patients. As discussed in Section 6.3, this "exposure-matching" strategy relies upon the condition/assumption that the disease pathobiology, mechanism of action of drug product, and the exposure–response relationships for both efficacy and safety are similar between pediatric and adult patients.

One recent example in the pediatric oncology domain was daunorubicin and cytarabine liposome injection, for treatment of newly diagnosed therapy-related acute myeloid leukemia (t-AML) or AML with myelodysplasia-related changes (AML-MRC) in pediatric patients of 1 year and older. The approval was based on finding of a survival benefit demonstrated in adult study with extrapolation of the efficacy to the pediatric population. PK, activity, and safety data in pediatrics were available from two single-arm trials, which included patients in the following age groups: seven patients of 1 year to less than 2 years old, 33 patients of 2 years to less than 12 years old, and 13 patients of 12 years old to less than 17 years old. No new safety signals were observed in pediatric patients in these two single-arm trials. No differences in safety were observed by age. The etiopathogeneses and natural histories of t-AML and of AML-MRC are essentially the same in adult and pediatric patients. Additionally, the approach to standard-of-care therapy for AML is also the same for adult and pediatric patients with AML, since there is no known difference in sensitivity of the AML cells to chemotherapy based on age rather than mutation profile. In exposure–response analyses, cytarabine exposure was a significant covariate for clinical activity and safety outcomes, but age was not significant, further supporting the extrapolation and appropriateness of exposure matching. Lastly, the population PK models based on data from pediatric and adult patients confirmed that the recommended dose provided appropriate exposure of total daunorubicin and cytarabine in pediatric patients which were comparable to the observed values in adults. These data provide substantial evidence to support extrapolation of efficacy from the adult indication, and the recommended dose for the pediatric population of 1 year and older (FDA, 2021b).

6.4.2 Dose Optimization

Conducting extensive dose-finding studies for optimal dose selection is challenging in rare disease, particularly in the pediatric population. However, well-planned drug development programs are often able to leverage the MIDD approaches to maximize the information generated for decision-making. There are various cases where model-based analyses, supplemented by the totality of evidence from the nonclinical and clinical development programs, served as the primary evidence for approval of untested dosing regimen in the pediatric population. Typically, recommending an untested dosing regimen instead of the studied one was to further optimize the benefit/risk profile, and/or to improve adherence/reduced complexity in treatment administration (Wang et al., 2019).

The example of adalimumab in pediatric ulcerative colitis (UC) was for both purposes. Adalimumab injection was approved in 2021 for the treatment of moderately to severely active UC in pediatric patients of 5 years of age and older weighing 20 kg and above. The effectiveness was demonstrated in a randomized, double-blind trial in 93 pediatric patients 5–17 years of age. Two levels of body weight-based (mg/kg) dosing regimen were evaluated, and better efficacy was observed in patients receiving the higher dosage during the 52-week trial. The final recommended dosing regimen differs from what was studied in the pediatric UC trial in multiple aspects, including a switch from mg/kg-based dosing regimen to body weight-tiered fixed doses, changes in dosing schedule, and adding an option of less frequent dosing regimen for the maintenance. This recommended dosing regimen was derived based on exposure bridging strategy with both efficacy and safety considerations. Specifically, it was selected through popPK modeling and simulation to provide adequate exposure in patients with varying body weight, that was associated with the studied higher dosage and better efficacy in the pediatric UC trial, while within the observed safe range from other adult and pediatric trials. The safety profile of adalimumab has been widely established in multiple indications in adults and pediatrics, with no apparent exposure–safety relationship identified in adult or pediatric populations (FDA, 2021a).

6.4.3 Clinical Trial Design

Another area for the application of MIDD in drug development for pediatric rare disease is informing clinical trial design. In the 2017 FDA Guidance for Industry "Pediatric Rare Diseases—A Collaborative Approach for Drug Development using Gaucher Disease as a Model", it is encouraged that whenever new studies in children are deemed necessary, modeling and simulation should be used to optimize pediatric studies (e.g., design, sample size, starting doses, timing of sampling, and number of samples) and particularly to inform the dosing rationale (https://www.fda.gov/regulatory-information/search-fda-guidance-documents/pediatric-rare-diseases-collaborative-approach-drug-development-using-gaucher-disease-model-draft).

In pediatric trials, optimization of the sampling strategy is often important for minimizing the number of patients and blood sampling required. Clinical trial simulation can help design the optimal PK sampling windows to minimize number of blood samples, add flexibility to timing of sample collection while ensuring robust estimates of the PK parameters.

For many diseases, disease progression models are being developed to understand the natural history of these diseases specifically in identifying influential baseline factors, important biomarkers for disease progression, characterizing endpoints, and duration with the aim of understanding likelihood of success. In the case of childhood-onset dystrophinopathy, associations between genetic mutations and loss of ambulation (LoA) were quantified in male patients to understand variation in disease progression which may be useful for clinical trial design (Haber et al., 2020). In this research, Haber et al. analyzed genetic and clinical data from the Muscular Dystrophy Surveillance, Tracking, and Research Network for 358 males born and diagnosed from 1982 to 2011. Genetic mutations were defined by overall type (deletion/duplication/point mutation) and among deletions, those amenable to exon-skipping therapy (exons 8, 20, 44–46 51–53) and another group. Cox proportional hazards regression modeling identified that exons 8 (HR=0.22; 95% CI=0.08, 0.63) and 44 (HR=0.30; 95% CI=0.12, 0.78) were associated with delayed LoA compared to other exon deletions. Mutation type did not predict time to LoA. These findings suggest that clinical trials including exons 8 and 44 skippable males should consider mutation information prior to randomization.

6.4.4 Summary

Given the practical and ethical challenges in drug development for pediatric rare disease, model-informed approaches leveraging all available information (e.g., disease, drug, placebo effect, PK/PD in nonclinical and clinical settings) are powerful and should be applied whenever appropriate to facilitate decision-making. To ensure the appropriate use of MIDD given the complexity and potential uncertainty, important considerations should also be taken ahead, including the context of use and risk, the extent and quality of the existing knowledge, and validity of underlying assumptions. A learn-and-confirm approach is commonly recommended, for newly available data to be used to confirm predictions as well as to continuously develop and improve the models.

6.5 Bayesian Approach

As discussed in Section 6.2, typically, evidence-based regulatory standards for approvals of medicines are the same for adult and pediatric patients. The ideal requirements are in general from adequate and well-controlled investigations. However, conducting clinical trials in children has many challenges, from biological and societal to economic. Recognizing the challenges, both the Food and Drug Administration (FDA) in US and the EMA have explored methods to authorize the use of new medicines through data extrapolation from adult clinical trials (Pellock et al., 2012).

Wadsworth, Hampson, and Jaki (2018) searched the web of science to identify statistical methods that could be used to support partial or no extrapolation in pediatric drug development programs prior to January 31, 2014. They have identified 102 methods comprising 58 Bayesian and 44 frequentist approaches. Similar search has been conducted by the pediatric subteam of the Drug Information Association Bayesian Scientific Working Group and Adaptive Design Working Group on Bayesian extrapolation of adult clinical trial information in pediatric drug evaluation (Gamalo-Siebers et al., 2017). In this section, the Bayesian approaches found to be useful in the pediatric program are discussed.

6.5.1 Background on Bayesian Statistics

Extrapolation is to extend information and conclusions available from studies in one or more subgroups of the patient population (the *source* population) to make inferences for another subgroup of the population (the *target* population) (EMA, 2018). By proper extrapolation, it can reduce the need to generate additional information to reach conclusions for the target population for ethical reasons, feasibility restrictions, or efficacy, to allow resources be allocated to areas where studies are the most needed (Gamalo-Siebers et al., 2017).

Frequentist statistical approaches to evaluate investigational drugs' efficacy and safety require relatively large number of patients, powered to detect a clinically meaningful treatment difference. Each investigational drug needs to establish its efficacy and safety on its own without combining information from external sources. In contrast, Bayesian statistical methods permit the combining of information from disparate sources.

To allow properly combining information in Bayesian methods, Gamalo-Siebers et al., (2017) described the requirements for optimal pediatric development plan when considering borrowing from adult, and the idea can be generalized to combine other types of source population with target population (pediatrics):

1. Understand the disease in question, the similarity between adults and children, and its incidence and prevalence in children.

2. Understand the expected treatment response differences in children, if any.

3. Allow the possibility of borrowing information from previous studies (adult and pediatrics) and specify the proper extent of the borrowing, determined by study quality or the similarity of the various data sources and expert opinion.

4. Optimize trial sample size through better use of prior data while maintaining adequate study power and monitoring type I error rate.

In Bayesian framework, the prior distribution refers to the distribution of our prior expectation on the investigational drug to work in the target population with the knowledge of the source population, and the posterior distribution is our updated estimate as the data from the trial are prospectively accumulated.

Denote θ as the target parameter to evaluate an investigational drug. For example, for pediatric cancer, θ is typically the objective response rate, that is, the proportion of patients responding to the investigational drug. Let D be the observed clinical trial data. The likelihood of θ given D is denoted by $L(\theta \mid D)$. Instead of maximizing this function to find the most probable estimation of θ, Bayesian methods add a *prior* distribution $\pi(\theta)$ to summarizing what is known about the parameter θ before the trial data D are collected. The prior may be based on a variety of sources: historical observational data, adult or older age group clinical trial data, data from the class of drugs with the same mechanism of action or auxiliary information such as expert clinical opinion, or taken as noninformative, which indicates no information is relevant and the prior would vanish from calculation. A Bayesian then computes the posterior distribution $p(\theta \mid D)$ via Bayes rule (Bayes, 1765) using either probability calculation or where closed-form calculations are not possible, a numerical approach such as MCMC (Carlin and Louis, 2009).

6.5.2 General Methods

As described, formal proof of efficacy of a new drug is obtained by using additional information (data, opinion, or expectation) expressed through a prior distribution. The impact of the prior assumptions on the evaluation of outcome and prespecified strategies for decision-making is required in the regulatory context. Noninformative prior distributions usually do not change the conclusions irrespective of the chosen analysis methods, while informative prior distributions would (Weber et al., 2018). The following discussion would describe the two categories of the prior distributions separately.

6.5.2.1 Noninformative Priors

Noninformative priors or reference priors are intended to provide a kind of distribution that is free from subjectivity (Spiegelhalter et al., 2004).

Commonly used noninformative prior distribution is uniform or flat prior. A uniform or flat prior means that all values of θ are equally likely; therefore, the posterior distribution has the same shape as likelihood function, which in turn means that the results of Bayesian intervals and estimations will match the frequentist results.

Alternatively, Jeffreys' prior can be used where any rule for determining the prior distribution should yield an equivalent result if applied to the transformed parameter (Jeffreys, 1961). For example, if a reference prior on an odds ratio (OR) should be the same whichever treatment is taken in the numerator of the odds ratio, then it means that the same prior should hold for OR and 1/OR, which implies uniform distribution on log(OR) scale.

Essentially, when noninformative prior is applied, there is no borrowing or combining information with the target population. The estimation and the inference of the outcome in pediatric is the same as the pediatric trial itself.

6.5.2.2 Informative Priors

A common challenge for drug development in rare diseases and pediatric population is the small numbers of patients that can be recruited into clinical trials. Utilization of available sources of information would be crucial for feasibility to establish efficacy evidence of investigational drug in pediatrics. Formally incorporating available sources of information would create an informative prior in Bayesian approaches. Wadsworth et al. (2018) identified 58 Bayesian methods from 25 papers. Of these, 54 methods created an informative prior while four assessed the consistency of treatment effects or PK responses between the source and target populations.

The methods to create informative priors can generally be categorized in Table 6.1. The numbers in the table are the number of methods reported in each category (Wadsworth et al., 2018). Difference between source population and target population can attribute to different relevant factors including but not limited to the following: dissimilar between adult and pediatric population, patient management or standards of care, trial protocols, demographic shifts in population over time, and operator training/experience. Therefore, majority of the methods discount the source data to account the potential differences except eight methods (Wadsworth et al., 2018). If there is no discounting, the informative prior $\pi(\theta)$ is created from source population and the final posterior distribution for source population would attribute equal weight to the source and target population data; therefore, source population

TABLE 6.1

Method Categories for Informative Prior and Combine with Trial Data

	Dynamic/Adaptive Borrowing	Fixed/Nonadaptive Borrowing
Discount from source	31	15
No discount from source	8	

is pooled with target trial data D without downweighting to derive a posterior distribution $p(\theta|D, D_S) \propto \pi(\theta) L(\theta|D, D_S)$, where D_S denotes the source population data.

In Gamalo-Siebers et al. (2017), they referred the nonadaptive borrowing as two-step approach. The two-step approach would calculate the posterior of the source population supplemental data (in their paper adult data) before combining with the trial data. The dynamic borrowing is referred as combined approaches or partial exchangeability approach in Gamalo-Siebers et al., (2017), and the partial exchangeability approach would be equivalent to discount from source with dynamic borrowing in Table 6.1.

Wadsworth, Hampson, and Jaki (2018) categorized the methods with its variations together. For example, they separated power prior with ten variations as 11 different methods. The variations of the methods can be able to shift the location and/or inflate the standard error of an estimate. For the purpose of discussing general methods, we focus on the main methodologies in this chapter.

6.5.2.2.1 Discount from Source and Nonadaptive Borrowing Methodologies

The power prior (Ibrahim et al., 2015) is a useful class of informative priors for historical borrowing. The goal is to downweight the historical data to some degree via a power $\alpha_0 \in [0,1]$. Use the same notations of the prior distribution as $\pi(\theta)$, source population data D_S, and the posterior distribution is calculated as $p(\theta|D, D_S, \alpha_0) \propto \pi(\theta) L(\theta|D_S)^{\alpha_0} L(\theta|D)$. When $\alpha_0 = 0$, there is no borrowing from source population, and when $\alpha_0 = 1$, there is full borrowing. Any number between 0 and 1 controls how much information will be borrowed from the source data to supplement the target population pediatric trial.

The mixture prior is another useful class of informative priors. Use the descriptions in Ye et al. (2020), the mixed prior is formulated as $\pi(\theta|D_S, a) = (1-a) f(D_S) + a G(D_S)$, where $G(D_S)$ is the enthusiastic prior distribution (e.g., source data D_S reflect pediatric data), $f(D_S)$ is either skeptical prior distribution (e.g., source data D_S are completely different from pediatric data and minimal response expected in pediatric patients) or noninformative distribution, and the relevance factor $a = \Pr(\text{applicability of source data})$. When $a = 0$ or 0%, the prior distribution indicates 0% applicability of the source data, that is, no borrowing. When $a = 1$ or 100%, the prior distribution indicates 100% applicability of the source data, that is, full borrowing. A number in between 0 and 1 corresponds to the amount of information borrowed from the source data. The posterior distribution is updated as $p(\theta|D, D_S, a) \propto \pi(\theta|D_S, a) L(\theta|D)$.

Both class of priors are nonadaptive because the control parameter α_0 or a is predetermined from source data as fixed and combine with the target pediatric population. Several authors discussed how to determine the control parameter. De Santis (2006) defines the power prior $\alpha_0 = r/n_S$, where n_S

is the sample size from the source population and r is a constant specified by the analyst. When there is more than one historical dataset from the source population, the weights will be given to different datasets in their relevance to the new target trial. Rietbergen et al. (2011) assign the control parameter from each historical study a weight elicited from expert opinion.

Other methods are available. Schoenfeld et al. (2009) augment data from a clinical trial in children with data from completed adult trial(s). The prior distribution is specified as $N(\theta^*, \sigma^2)$. The choice of the parameter can be derived from opinion between population differences or derived from a meta-analysis of adult studies. Chen et al. (2009) derive a Bayesian empirical prior distribution for target treatment effect in a local region of a multi-regional clinical trial using normal distribution $\pi(\theta) \sim N(\hat{\mu}, \sigma^2)$. The $\hat{\mu}$ is determined as global treatment effect estimate by averaging the effect estimates across each region; therefore, the target regional treatment effect borrows strength from data in other regions. The σ^2 is taken to be a linear function of the variance of the region-specific effect estimates, where smaller values of the coefficient of the interregional variance allow for more borrowing of strength across regions. The authors recommend the coefficient to be prespecified to reflect the consensus opinion of local regulatory authority and trial sponsor.

6.5.2.2.2 *Sensitivity of Priors*

When there is control parameter in the informative prior, the robustness of the informative priors can be evaluated based on sensitivity analysis. By varying the control parameter in the informative priors, the robustness of the posterior distribution can be plotted against the control parameter to show when the decision based on posterior distribution would change.

6.5.2.2.3 *Discount from Source and Adaptive Borrowing Methodologies*

In 2016, US FDA Center for Devices and Radiological Health (CDRH) issued a guidance and promotion on hierarchical models to be used in pediatric extrapolation in medical devices (US Food and Drug Administration (FDA), 2016). In a hierarchical model, a common distribution is assumed across studies (target population and source population) with an explicit parameter τ measuring the variation across studies. A prior distribution is placed on τ that is then updated using the current data. A discrepancy between the source and target population would put more weight toward larger τ values in the posterior distribution than would an agreement between the source and target populations. Therefore, the borrowing depends on τ and incorporates its uncertainty, producing dynamic borrowing (Viele et al., 2014).

Use our notations in the chapter. Denote the prior distribution as $\pi(\theta)$ and source population data D_S with parameter $\theta_S = \{\theta_{S_1}, ..., \theta_{S_k}\}$, $k = 1, ..., K$ if there are more than one source population data. In a hierarchical model, θ and θ_{S_k} are indistinguishable (i.e., exchangeable), then there exists a distribution G such that $\theta, \theta_{S_k} \mid \xi \sim G(\xi), \xi \sim H(\tau)$, where the second-stage prior distribution (or hyperprior) H describes the initially available information about ξ, i.e., $H(\tau) = \pi(\xi) = \pi(\mu \mid \tau^2)\pi(\tau^2)$ and τ measures the between-study variability. For simplicity, if $G \sim N(\mu, \tau^2)$ with $\xi = (\mu, \tau^2)$, the exchangeability of the parameters in source and target population data means $\theta, \theta_{S_1}, ..., \theta_{S_k} \mid \mu, \tau^2 \sim N(\mu, \tau^2)$; thus, they have a common mean μ and between-study variability τ^2. The key parameter τ. controls the borrowing. For $\tau \approx 0$, it is extremely likely that all the θ_{S_k} will be similar (thus borrowing extensively would be appropriate), while for large τ, different source data may be quite different (and thus minimal borrowing is appropriate). Since we do not typically know μ, τ^2, the hyper prior distributions are placed on μ, τ^2, creating a hierarchical structure, for example, hyperprior distributions with $\mu \sim N(\mu_0, \tau_0), \tau^2 \sim IGamma(\alpha, \beta)$. When combine the source population data with our target population data, the joint posterior distribution based on hierarchical model would be $p(\theta, \theta_S, \tau^2 \mid D_S) \propto \pi(\tau^2)\pi(\theta_S, \theta \mid \tau^2)\, L(\theta, \theta_S, \tau^2 \mid D_S)$.

When source data and target data may be dissimilar (e.g., adult supplemental data and the pediatric data), partial exchangeability approach can be utilized. This is by adding additional layer to the hierarchical model that expressed nonexchangeability: $\theta_{S_{jk}} \big| \xi_j \sim G(\xi_j), \xi_j \big| \tau \sim H(\tau), \tau \sim P$. Here $\theta_{S_{jk}}$ denotes the parameter of source data from the kth study within the jth population (e.g., adult or pediatric). Conditional on the population covariate level or within each population j, the studies are exchangeable, but not across populations. For the example of adult as source population and pediatric as target population, the posterior distribution would be: $p(\xi_{\text{peds}}, \theta_S, \xi_{\text{adult}}, \tau \mid D, D_S) \propto L(\theta_{\text{peds}} \mid D)L(\theta_{\text{adult}} \mid D_S)\pi(\theta)\pi(\xi_{\text{peds}})\pi(\xi_{\text{adult}})\pi(\tau)$, where $\theta = (\theta_{\text{peds}}, \theta_{\text{adult}})$ (Gamalo-Siebers et al., 2017).

Another class of method to combine data across several heterogeneous source populations to formulate an informative prior is meta-analytic predictive (MAP) priors. The models are formulated assuming source population historical data D_S and target contemporary data D are exchangeable. Denote $\theta_S = \{\theta_{S_1}, ..., \theta_{S_k}\}$, $k = 1, ..., K$ as the source population parameters if there are more than one source population data. In derivation of the MAP priors, Neuenschwander et al. (2010) assumed the source clinical trials $D_S = \{D_{S_1}, ..., D_{S_k}\}$ follow normal distribution, for example, $D_{S_k} \mid \theta_{S_k} \sim N(\theta_{S_k}, S_{S_k})$ and known standard errors $S_S = \{S_{S_1}, ..., S_{S_k}\}$. The MAP model is to synthesize data from the control arms of the historical source data in a Bayesian random-effects meta-analytical model to derive the posterior predictive distribution for the target population of interest in the control group of the new study. Therefore, the Bayesian random-effects meta-analytical model can be written as follows: $\theta_{S_1}, ..., \theta_{S_k}, \theta \mid \mu, \tau^2 \sim N(\mu, \tau^2)$, $\mu \sim \pi(\mu), \tau^2 \sim \pi(\tau^2)$. In the special case that τ^2 is known, the posterior predictive distribution given the historical source data is as follows: $p(\theta \mid D_S, \tau^2) \sim N\left(\dfrac{\sum w_k D_{S_k}}{\sum w_k}, \dfrac{1}{\sum w_k} + \tau^2\right),$

where $w_k = \left(S_{S_k}^2 + \tau\right)^{-1}$. When τ^2 is unknown, the authors recommend use priors on τ^2 that puts most of the distribution on values that represent plausible heterogeneity and less probability to the unanticipated heterogeneity.

Similar to the discussion in hierarchical model, when there can be conflict between historical source data and target contemporary data, the similarity of parameters is violated. Instead of using the hierarchical model to derive the prior, alternatively, robust MAP priors can be derived. Schmidli et al. (2014) proposed the prior to be specified as a weighted average between MAP-prior $\theta_{S_{MAP}}$. (derived same as above) and a weakly informative prior: $\pi(\theta|w) = (1-w)\pi(\text{Weakly} - \text{informative}) + w\pi(\theta_{S_{MAP}})$, where w controls the prior probability that the source data are relevant for the target population, similar to the relevant factor of probability of applicability in mixture prior. The determination of w is typically prespecified, and similar consideration in mixture prior applies.

Hobbs et al. (2011) adjust the power prior parameter through a measure of the degree to which the historical data and current data are commensurate; therefore, the borrowing is adaptive based on commensurability and attenuation occurs when it is appropriate. Use the same notations $\pi(\theta_S)$ as prior distribution, source population data D_S, and the posterior distribution is calculated as $p(\theta,\theta_S|D,D_S,\tau) \propto \pi(\theta_S)\pi(\tau)\pi(\theta|\theta_S,D_S,\tau)L(\theta_S|D_S)L(\theta|D) \propto \pi(\theta|D_S,\theta_S,\tau)L(\theta|D)$, where τ is introduced as commensurate parameter and is inversely related to the between-study variance parameter for the random-effects meta-analytic models and $\pi(\theta_S)$ reflects (typically vague) initial prior knowledge about θ_S before seeing D_S. Normal commensurate prior is usually used since it most conveniently captures between-study variability through τ and its hyper prior. When τ approaches 0, $\pi(\theta|D_S,\theta_S,\tau) \to \pi(\theta_S)$, effectively ignoring the source data. On the other hand, as $\tau \to \infty$, θ approaches θ_S and $\pi(\theta|D_S,\theta_S,\tau) \to L(\theta|D_S)\pi(\theta_S)$, the prior assumes full commensurability of the target and source data by pooling them together.

6.5.3 Effective Sample Size

The amount of information borrowed from source data through the construction of the prior distribution is quantified as effective sample size (ESS). When using conjugate priors for the exponential family, the ESS is easily obtained (Bernardo and Smith, 2000). For example, if prior distribution is chosen to be $\pi(\theta) \sim Beta(a,b)$ and the trial data follow binomial distribution $D(x,N,\theta) = \text{Binomial}(N,\theta)$, this beta-binomial model would give the conjugate posterior distribution $Beta(a+x,b+N-x)$. The total ESS is $a+b+N$ and includes a gain of $a+b$ effective patients from prior distribution; therefore, the ESS is $a+b$. Based on the observation, Morita et al. (2008) proposed a definition for the ESS as the value to minimize the "prior-to-posterior" distance. They define an ε-information prior $\pi_b(\theta)$ as a prior having the same parametric family and mean as $\pi(\theta)$ but with arbitrarily large variance; therefore,

$\pi_b(\theta)$ is a prior with prior ESS approximately equal to zero. The ESS is calculated as minimizing the difference between the posterior distribution induced by the prior $\pi_b(\theta)$ and the trial data and the information contained in the prior $\pi(\theta)$ (Wiesenfarth & Calderazzo, 2020). An alternative heuristic formula introduced by Malec (2001) is to calculate ESS based on the ratio of the posterior variance in the study without borrowing from prior studies, to the posterior variance in the study with borrowing, multiplied by the study sample size (Gamalo-Siebers et al., 2017).

When prior distribution from source population and trial data for target pediatric population conflict, Reimherr et al. (2014) proposed an algorithm comparing two posteriors, rather than a prior and a posterior, to measure the information. Wiesenfarth and Calderazzo (2020) further extend to define effective current sample size (ECSS) to minimize the distance in mean square error (MSE) between the posterior mean estimate induced by the prior $\pi(\theta)$ and the trial data and the posterior mean estimate by the prior $\pi_b(\theta)$ and the trial data. In other words, the information contained in a posterior is the sum of the information contained in the prior and in the likelihood. The ECSS quantifies the number of samples to be added or subtracted to the posterior if the informative prior and trial data are in sync or in conflict, respectively.

6.5.4 Operating Characteristics

When Bayesian approach is used in pediatric labeling, regulatory agencies can request the operating characteristics be assessed for proposed data combination procedures and especially those involving multiple testing. As discussed in Gamalo-Siebers et al. (2017), even though evaluating expected type I and type II error rates is at odds with Bayesian approach, it is generally considered good statistical practice to evaluate the frequentist operating characteristics. The corresponding type I error rate in Bayesian approach is the probability of observing study (target pediatric) data and prior (source population) data that together falsely reject the null hypothesis, as averaged over the variability in both the unknown parameters and the as-yet unobserved data. For example, if the Bayesian decision rule is to reject the null hypothesis when $P(\delta > 0 \mid D, D_s) \geq p^*$, where δ is the treatment difference and p^* is a prespecified threshold value, we seek a model and prior such that the rate of this decision is less than some upper bound $\alpha \in (0,1)$, maximized over the variability of unknown parameters and as-yet unobserved data D, when there is indeed no difference.

Similarly, the corresponding type II error or 1-power in Bayesian approach is the probability of observing study (target pediatric) data and prior (source population) data that together unable to reject the null hypothesis when there is treatment difference, as averaged over the variability in both the unknown parameters and the as-yet unobserved data. For example, the frequentist equivalent Bayesian type II error can be calculated as $1 - P(\delta > 0 \mid D, D_s) \geq p^\#$, where δ is the treatment difference and $p^\#$ is a prespecified threshold value, and we seek a model and prior such that the rate of this decision is less than some upper bound $\beta \in (0,1)$, maximized over the variability of unknown parameters and as-yet unobserved data D, when there is treatment difference.

6.5.5 Decision Rule

As discussed in Section 6.5.4, the decision rule using Bayesian approach would be made based on posterior probability. If target parameter in pediatric population θ is assumed to test the null hypothesis as $H_0 : \theta \le 0$ against the alternative $H_1 : \theta > 0$. Then, the decision rule is based on the posterior probability $p(\theta > 0 | D, D_S) > 1 - c/2$, for some threshold $1 - c/2$. If the threshold is 0.975, the $c = 0.05$. For time-to-event endpoints (or ratios), the target parameter is to test the null hypothesis of hazard ratio (or odds ratio) as $H_0 : \theta \le 1$ against the alternative $H_1 : \theta > 1$. Similarly, the posterior probability is calculated $p(\theta > 1 | D, D_S) > 1 - c/2$. The threshold should be calibrated so that the desired type I error is achieved. The desired type I error may not necessarily be 0.025 and should be discussed and agreed with regulatory agencies given that there generally is limited pediatric and rare disease population and high unmet medical.

6.5.6 Case Example

We illustrate one example that borrowed adult approval data to construct an informative prior and combine with pediatric trial data to inform the pediatric efficacy. This example is described in more details in Ye et al. (2020). CML is a rare cancer, occurring between 1 and 1.5 cases per 100,000 (National Institute of Health (NIH), 2020). Nilotinib was approved by the US FDA in 2018 to treat pediatric patients greater than 1 year of age with newly diagnosed Philadelphia chromosome-positive CML (Ph+ CML) in chronic phase, which is a subset of CML. Table 6.2 summarizes the clinical trial designs and results of the primary endpoint MMR at 12 months used in the approval of nilotinib for the treatment of newly diagnosed Ph+ CML in chronic phase. The approval in adults was based on a randomized clinical trial, where patients were randomized 1:1 to treat with either nilotinib or imatinib with sample size of 282 and 283, respectively. The pediatric approval was based on a single-arm study with 25 patients.

TABLE 6.2

Comparison of Adult and Pediatric Approval of Nilotinib

	Adult	Pediatric
Design	Randomized	Single-arm
Sample size	Nilotinib $N=282$ versus imatinib $N=283$	$N=25$
Age	18+	2–18
MMR at 12 months[a]	44% (38.4, 50.3)	60% (38.7, 78.9)

[a] Results are for primary endpoint, for other information refer to USPI.

A mixture prior for response rate θ was constructed as $\pi(\theta| D_S,a) = (1-a)f(D_S)+aG(D_S)$, where a is 50% indicating adult data are 50% relevant to the pediatric study. The $G(D_S)$ is enthusiastic/adult prior Beta(8,13) and centered at response rate at about 38%, slightly discounted from adult approval data with ESS of 21 patients. It places low probability of observing response rate less than 20% (2.5% chance). The $f(D_S)$ is skeptical prior as Beta(1.2, 12) with ESS of 13.2 patients, which centers at response rate roughly 9%, indicating no meaningful clinical benefit. The probability to observe a high response rate, for example, over 30%, is 2.5%.

Suppose 30% response rate is considered minimally clinically meaningful in this population. We consider efficacy to be defined as the probability of MMR rate greater than 30% in pediatrics. The posterior distribution using the mixture prior combined with pediatric clinical trial data would give $p(\theta \geq 30\%| D,D_S,a = 50\%) = 99.7\%$, indicating high probability of efficacy in pediatric patients.

A sensitivity analysis was conducted by varying the control parameter a from 5% to 100% with increment of 5%. Even with 5% applicability of adult study, the posterior probability is greater than 98%. The result is very robust to the choice of probability of applicability and shows strong support for efficacy in pediatric group in this case example.

6.6 Other Aspects and Discussions

6.6.1 Neonates and Preterm Babies

Neonates and preterm babies represent a unique challenge in drug development programs. There are significant physiological changes in fetus during utero development involving the normal expression and maturation of organs and tissues including enzyme systems, receptors, transporters, and neurotransmitters. Most drugs used in neonatal intensive care units (NICUs) are off-label; therefore, it is important that drug studies be conducted in neonates to address gaps in pediatric labeling information (US Food and Drug Administration (FDA), 2019f). Leveraging knowledge and data obtained from adult, preclinical and other pediatric studies coupled with quantitative approaches such as population pharmacokinetics (PopPK), and PBPK modeling can help predict neonatal doses and optimal clinical trial design. When designing studies, consider stratifying the neonatal population to decrease heterogeneity. Gestational age (GA) at birth, postnatal age (PNA), and other factors (e.g., concurrent illness and underlying disease) are all important stratification factors. Since blood samples are the primary samples collected in neonatal studies, the volumes needed should be limited to the least possible and follow the institutional guidelines for total blood volume limits for neonatal studies. Sparse sampling utilizing opportunistic sampling and the use of scavenged samples is a practical approach to increase the feasibility to obtain pharmacokinetic data (US Food and Drug Administration (FDA), 2019f).

Unique considerations should be made for age-appropriate dosage formulation in neonates. All aspects of the formulation, including the salt forms of the active ingredient, the excipients, and the volume of the unit dose (especially permit the accurate dosing of potentially small unit doses), should be considered. Additionally, alternative route of administration, including but not limited to enteral, inhalational, intraocular, transcutaneous, intramuscular, subcutaneous, or rectal, can be considered when appropriate. Minimize the use of excipients in neonatal formulations whenever possible given that the accumulation of excipients may be significantly higher in neonates due to immature organ function. Excipients with known toxicity in neonates should not be used (e.g., ethanol, propylene glycol, benzyl alcohol) (US Food and Drug Administration (FDA), 2019f).

6.6.2 Data Quality, Collection, and Sharing

Given the rarity of the disease, integrating data from existing rare disease data collections including registries, clinical trials, observational studies, and natural history studies can be valuable to accelerate research and aid drug development. But since the data are from diverse sources across a multitude of rare diseases, different organizations, and different types of studies, integration of patient-level data presents unique challenges. The Rare Disease Cures Accelerator-Data and Analytics Platform (RDCA-DAP) is an FDA-funded initiative that provides a centralized and standardized infrastructure to promote the sharing of existing patient-level data and encourages the standardization of new data collection (Critical Path Institute, 2020). In Europe, the European Platform on Rare Disease Registration (EU RD Platform) has similar objectives to enable integration of various registries across Europe and to maximize the value of each registry and data collection, standardization, and exchange of new registries (European Commission, 2020). By establishing public–private partnership to enable analyzing shared patient-level data, it can help create solutions to many challenges in the medical product development. Examples include but are not limited to the following: including placebo response in disease trial model, stage-specific outcome measures based on quantitative disease progression model, quantification of disease progression as a function of biomarker status prior to diagnosis, quantification of disease progression as a function of baseline characteristics, enrichment biomarker, model-based biomarker qualification and stratification of patient populations, clinical trial simulation tool based on disease trial model and value of use of historical controls, qualification and validation of outcome measures, and qualification of prognostic biomarker (Karpen et al., 2021).

6.6.3 Animal Rule

Under rare circumstances, US regulations known as animal rule (Regulations, 2002) can be applied to support the approval of the drugs and biological products when human efficacy studies are not ethical and field trials to study the effectiveness are not feasible. Under the animal rule, the efficacy is established based on adequate and well-controlled studies in animal models of human disease or condition of interest. The safety is evaluated under the pre-existing requirements for drugs and biological products. For example, obiltoxaximab injection was approved in March 2016 based on animal rule. The approval included pediatric patients for treatment of inhalational anthrax due to *B. anthracis* in combination with appropriate antibacterial drugs, and for prophylaxis of inhalational anthrax when alternative therapies are not available or are not appropriate.

Over the past 50–60 years, great progress has been made in diagnosis, treatment, and survival of childhood cancer. In the 1960s, the probability of survival for a child with cancer was less than 25%, whereas today it may exceed 80%. The key principles contributing to the successful treatment of childhood cancer include the following:

- Recognition of the importance of timing of therapy and that different agents and intensity of therapy are required for different disease burdens,
- Tumor biology predicts clinical behavior,
- Development and evolution of staging systems that incorporate clinical, surgical, and biological features,
- Risk stratification to improve outcome and diminish morbidity,
- Use of preclinical models and underlying tumor biology to identify and test potential active agents,
- Pharmacokinetics and pharmacogenetic monitoring of anticancer drugs,
- Importance of supportive care, the child as a member of the family unit, and
- Establishment of cooperative groups/consortia and training and education of specialized professionals and recognition of cancer survival as a life continuum (McGregor et al., 2007).

Development of effective treatments for rare disease and in pediatric population poses unique scientific and ethical challenges in addition to the small markets. Even though not all principles contributed to the success of childhood cancers can be applicable to other rare pediatric diseases, certain aspects can be useful when implemented and progress has been made over the years. In this chapter, those interrelated aspects that can contribute to successful drug development of rare pediatric diseases were extensively discussed, including the global regulations and regulatory programs that promote rare disease and pediatric drug development, the role of natural history and patient advocacy, the applicability of preclinical and nonclinical models, considerations of pediatric extrapolation, the study designs that are useful when no or partial extrapolation is considered, key approaches and considerations in use of modeling and simulations to support, and useful Bayesian approaches. Examples of successful clinical development programs have been discussed in the chapter. With more education and implementation, we expect to see more success of effective treatments for rare diseases in pediatric beyond childhood cancers.

Acknowledgment

The authors want to thank Shetarra Walker and Martin Rose from office of new drugs, Jialu Zhang from office of biostatistics, and Snehal Samant from office of clinical pharmacology in CDER, FDA for their review of the case example. (FDA), U. F. (2018). *Larotrectinib, US Prescriber Information (USPI)*. Retrieved from https://www.accessdata.fda.gov/drugsatfda_docs/label/2018/211710s000lbl.pdf. The authors also want to thank members of Vertex Basket/Umbrella Work Group, including Chenghao Chu, Shiyao Liu, Yang Chen, Yaohua Zhang, Yiyue Lou, and Lei Gao.

References

Akula, A. Y., Meng, X., Reaman, G. H., Ma, L., Yuan, W., & Ye, J. (2021). A review of the experience with pediatric written requests issued for oncology drug products. *Pediatric Blood and Cancer*, 68(2): e28828.

Barone, A., Casey, D., McKee, A. E., & Reaman, G. H. (2019). Cancer drugs approved for use in children: Impact of legislative initiatives and future opportunities. *Pediatric Blood and Cancer*, 66(8): e27809.

Bavdekar, S. B. (2013). Pediatric clinical trials. *Perspectives in Clinical Research*, 4(1): 89–99.

Bayes, T. (1765). An essay towards solving a problem in the doctrine of chances. *Philosophical Transactions of the Royal Society of London*, 54(1763): 370–418.

Bazzano, A. T., Mangione-Smith, R., Schonlau, M., Suttorp, M., & Brook, R. H. (2009). Off-label prescribing to children in the United States outpatient setting. *Academic Pediatrics*, 9(2): 81–88.

Bernardo, J., & Smith, A. (2000). *Bayesian Theory*. Chichester: John Wiley & Sons Ltd.

Bi, Y., Liu, J., Li, L., Bhattaram, A., Bewernitz, M., Li, R.-J., ... & Wang, Y. (2019). Role of model-informed drug development in pediatric drug development, regulatory evaluation, and labeling. *Journal of Clinical Pharmacology*, 59(S1): S104–S111.

Carlin, B., & Louis, T. (2009). *Bayesian Methods for Data Analysis*, 3rd Edition. Boca Raton, FL: CRC Press.

Carpenter, J., & Kenward, M. (2013). *Multiple Imputation and Its Application*. Chichester: John Wiley & Sons. 345 pages, ISBN: 9780470740521.

CDC. (n.d.). *Principles of Epidemiology in Public Health Practice*. Retrieved from https://www.cdc.gov/csels/dsepd/ss1978/lesson1/section9.html

Chen, Y.-H., Wu, Y.-C., & Wang, M. (2009). A Bayesian approach to evaluating regional treatment effect in a multiregional trial. *Journal of Biopharmaceutical Statistics*, 19(5): 900–915.

Chuk, M. K., Mulugeta, Y., Roth-Cline, M., Mehrotra, N., & Reaman, G. H. (2017). Enrolling adolescents in disease/target-appropriate adult oncology clinical trials of investigational agents. *Clinical Cancer Research*, 23(1): 9–12.

Code of Federal Regulations (CFR). (2020). *Title 21CFR314.126 Adequate and Well-Controlled Studies*. Retrieved from https://www.accessdata.fda.gov/scripts/cdrh/cfdocs/cfcfr/cfrsearch.cfm?fr=314.126

Conroy, S., Choonara, I., Impicciatore, P., Mohn, A., Arnell, H., Rane, A., ... & van Den Ankar, J. (2000). Survey of unlicensed and off label drug use in paediatric wards in European countries. *British Medical Journal*, 320(7227): 79.

Conroy, S., Mcintyre, J., Choonara, I., & Hull, D. (1999). Unlicensed and off label drug use in neonates. *Archives of Disease in Childhood - Fetal and Neonatal Edition*, 80(2):F142.

Critical Path Institute. (2020). *Rare Disease Cures Accelerator-Data and Analytics Platform (RDCA-DAP)*. Retrieved from https://c-path.org/programs/rdca-dap/

Day, S., Jonker, A. H., Lau, L. P. L., Hilgers, R.-D., Irony, I., Larsson, K., Roes, K. C. B., & Stallard, N. (2018). Recommendations for the design of small population clinical trials. *Orphanet Journal of Rare Diseases*, 13, Article number: 195.

De Santis, F. (2006). Power priors and their use in clinical trials. *The American Statistician*, 60(2): 122–129.

Department of Health and Human Services (HHS). (1998). Regulations requiring manufacturers to assess the safety and effectiveness of new drugs and biological products in pediatric patients: Final rule. *Federal Register*, 63(231): 66631–66672.

EMA/FDA. (2021). *Common Commentary-EMA/FDA: Common Issues Requested for Discussion by the Respective Agency (EMA/PDCO and FDA) Concerning Paediatric Oncology Development Plans (Paediatric Investigation Plans (PIPs] and Initial Pediatric Study Plans [iPSPs])*. Retrieved from https://www.ema.europa.eu/en/documents/other/common-commentary-ema/fda-common-issues-requested-discussion-respective-agency-ema/pdco-fda-concerning-paediatric-oncology-development-plans-paediatric-investigation-plans-pips_en.pdf

European Commission. (2020). *European Platform on Rare Disease Registration*. Retrieved from https://eu-rd-platform.jrc.ec.europa.eu/_en

European Medicines Agency (EMA). (n.d.). *Paediatric Investigation Plans*. Retrieved from https://www.ema.europa.eu/en/human-regulatory/research-development/paediatric-medicines/paediatric-investigation-plans

European Medicines Agency (EMA). (2007). *Reflection Paper on Methodological Issues in Confirmatory Clinical Trials Planned with an Adaptive Design*. Retrieved from https://www.ema.europa.eu/en/documents/scientific-guideline/reflection-paper-methodological-issues-confirmatory-clinical-trials-planned-adaptive-design_en.pdf

European Medicines Agency (EMA). (2018). *Reflection Paper on the Use of Extrapolation in the Development of Medicines for Paediatrics*. Retrieved from https://www.ema.europa.eu/en/documents/scientific-guideline/adopted-reflection-paper-use-extrapolation-development-medicines-paediatrics-revision-1_en.pdf

FDA. (2021a). *US Prescribing Information (USPI), Humira*. Retrieved from https://www.accessdata.fda.gov/drugsatfda_docs/label/2021/125057s417lbl.pdf

FDA. (2021b). *US Prescribing Information (USPI), Vyxeos*. Retrieved from https://www.accessdata.fda.gov/drugsatfda_docs/label/2021/209401s006lbl.pdf

Food and Drug Administration Modernization Act of 1997 (n.d.). Pub L No. 105-115, S. and Best Pharmaceuticals for Children Act, Pub L No. 107-109 Stat 1408.

Gamalo-Siebers, M., Savic, J., Basu, C., Zhao, X., Gopalakrishnan, M., Gao, A., ... & Carlin, B. P. (2017). Statistical modeling for Bayesian extrapolation of adult clinical trial information in pediatric drug evaluation. *Pharmaceutical Statistics*, 16(4): 232–249.

General Principals EMA-FDA Parallel Scientific Advice (Human Medicinal Products). (2017). Retrieved from https://www.fda.gov/media/105211/download

Green, D. J., Liu, X. I., Hua, T., Burnham, J. M., Schuck, R., Pacanowski, M., ... & Zineh, I. (2018). Enrichment strategies in pediatric drug development: An analysis of trials submitted to the US Food and Drug Administration. *Clinical Pharmacology & Therapeutics*, 104(5), 1–6.

Haber, G., Conway, K. M., Paramsothy, P., Roy, A., Rogers, H., Ling, X., ... & Bhattaram, V. A. (2020). Association of genetic mutations and loss of ambulation in childhood-onset dystrophinopathy. *Muscle and Nerve*, https://doi.org/10.1002/mus.27113.

Hobbs, B., Carlin, B., Mandrekar, S., & Sargent, D. (2011). Hierarchical commensurate and power prior models for adaptive incorporation of historical information in clinical trials. *Biometrics*, 67(3):1047–1056.

Houghton, P., Morton, C., Tucker, C., Payne, D., Favours, E., Cole, C., ... & Smith, M. (2007). The pediatric preclinical testing program: description of models and early testing results. *Pediatric Blood and Cancer*, 79(7): 928–940.

Ibrahim, J., Chen, M.-H., Gwon, Y., & Chen, F. (2015). The power prior: Theory and applications. *Statistics in Medicine*, 34(28):3724–3749.

ICH. (2010a). *ICH M3(R2) Guidance for Industry: Nonclinical Safety Studies for the Conduct of Human Clinical Trials and Marketing Authorization for Pharmaceuticals*. Retrieved from https://www.fda.gov/media/71542/download

ICH. (2010b). *ICH S9 Guidance for Industry: Nonclinical Evaluation for Anticancer Pharmaceuticals*. Retrieved from https://www.fda.gov/media/73161/download

ICH. (2012). *ICH S6(R1) Guidance for Industry: S6 Addendum to Preclinical Safety Evaluation of Biotechnology-Derived Pharmaceuticals*. Retrieved from https://www.fda.gov/media/78034/download

ICH. (2018). *ICH S9 Nonclinical Evaluation for Anticancer Pharmaceuticals Questions and Answers Guidance for Industry*. Retrieved from https://www.fda.gov/media/100344/download

ICH. (2021). *ICH S11 Guidance for Industry: Nonclinical Safety Testing in Support of Development of Pediatric Pharmaceuticals.* Retrieved from https://www.fda.gov/media/148478/download

Jeffreys, H. (1961). *Theory of Probability,* 3rd Edition. Oxford: Clarendon Press.

Karpen, S. R., White, J., Mullin, A. P., O'Doherty, I., Hudson, L. D., Romero, K., ... & Larkindale, J. (2021). Effective data sharing as a conduit for advancing medical product development. *Therapeutic Innovation and Regulatory Science,* 55: 591–600.

Kurmasheva, R., & Houghton, P. (2016). Identifying novel therapeutic agents using xenograft models of pediatric cancer. *Cancer Chemotherapy and Pharmacology,* 78(2): 221–232.

Leighton, J., Saber, H., Reaman, G., & Pazdur, R. (2016). An FDA oncology view of juvenile animal studies in support of initial pediatric studies for anticancer drugs. *Regulatory Toxicology and Pharmacology,* 79: 142–143.

Lesko, L. J. (2021). Perspective on model-informed drug development. *Pharmacometrics and Systems Pharmacology.* https://doi.org/10.1002/psp4.12699.

Lim, J., Walley, R., Yuan, J., Liu, J., Dacral, A., Best, N., ... & Bowen, E. (2018). Minimizing patient burden through the use of historical subject-level data in innovative confirmatory clinical trials: review of methods and opportunities. *Therapeutic Innovation and Regulatory Science,* 52(5): 546–559.

Madabushi, R., Benjamin, J. M., Grewal, R., Pacanowski, M. A., Strauss, D. G., Wang, Y., ... & Zineh, I. (2019). The US Food and Drug Administration's model-informed drug development paired meeting pilot program: Early experience and impact. *Clinical Pharmacology and Therapeutics,* https://doi.org/10.1002/cpt.1457.

Malec, D. (2001). A Closer Look at combining data among a small number of binomial experiments. *Statistics in Medicine,* 20(12): 1811–1824.

McGregor, L. M., Metzger, M. L., Sanders, R., & Santana, V. M. (2007). Pediatric cancers in the new millennium: Dramatic progress, new challenges. *Oncology,* 21(7): 809.

Morita, S., Thall, P., & Muller, P. (2008). Determining the effective sample size of a parametric prior. *Biometrics,* 64(2): 595–602.

National Cancer Institute (NCI). (n.d.). *Natural History Study.* Retrieved from https://www.cancer.gov/publications/dictionaries/cancer-terms/def/natural-history-study

National Institute of Health (NIH). (2020). *Rare Diseases.* Retrieved from https://rare-diseases.info.nih.gov/diseases/6105/chronic-myeloid-leukemia

Neuenschwander, B., Capkun-Niggli, G., Branson, M., & Spiegelhalter, D. (2010). Summarizing historical information on controls in clinical trials. *Clinical Trials,* 7(1): 5–18.

Ollivier, C., Mulugeta, Y. L., Guggieri, L., Saint-Raymond, A., & Yao, L. (2019). Paediatric extrapolation: A necessary paradigm shift. *British Journal of Clinical Pharmacology,* 85(4): 675–679. doi: 10.1111/bcp.13809.

Pellock, J. M., Carman, W. J., Thygarajan, V., Daniels, T., Morris, D. L., & D'Cruz, O. (2012). Efficacy of antiepileptic drugs in adults predicts efficacy in children: A systematic review. *Neurology,* 79: 1482–1489.

Reaman, G., Stancato, L., Vassal, G., & Maris, J. M. (2020). Crossing oceans: Preclinical collaboration to improve pediatric drug development. *American Society of Clinical Oncology Educational Book,* 40: 1–8. doi: 10.1200/EDBK_278893.

Regulations, C.-C. O. (2002). *21 CFR 314.600-650 for drugs; 21 CFR 601.90-95 for Biologics.* Retrieved from https://www.accessdata.fda.gov/scripts/cdrh/cfdocs/cfcfr/cfrsearch.cfm?fr=314.600

Reimherr, M., Meng, X.-L., & Nicolae, D. (2014). Being an informed Bayesian: Assessing prior informativeness and prior-likelihood conflict. *arXiv e-prints, arXiv:1406.5958v1*.

Rietbergen, C., Klugkist, I., Janssen, K., Moons, K., & Hoijtink, H. (2011). Incorporation of historical data in the analysis of randomized therapeutic trials. *Contemporary Clinical Trials*, 32: 848–855.

Ristovska, L. (2020). *Regulations and Data Sources on Pediatric Clinical Studies in the United States and European Union*. Retrieved from https://www.nber.org/sites/default/files/2020-08/Regulations%20and%20Data%20Sources%20on%20Pediatric%20Clinical%20Studies%20in%20the%2CUnited%20States%20and%20European%20Union.pdf

Rokita, J., Rathi, K., Cardenas, M., Upton, K. A., Jayaseelan, J., Cross, K. L., ... & Maris, J. M. (2019). Genomic profiling of childhood tumor patient-derived xenograft models to enable rational clinical trial design. *Cell Reports*, 29(6): 1675–1689.

Roth-Cline, M., & Nelson, R. (2014). The ethical principle of scientific necessity in pediatric research. *The American Journal of Bioethics*, 14(12):14–15.

Schmidli, H., Gseiger, S., Roychoudbury, S., O'Hagan, A., Spiegelhalter, D., & Neuenschwander, B. (2014). Robust meta-analytic-predictive priors in clinical trials with historical control information. *Biometrics*, 70(4): 1023–1032.

Schoenfeld, D., Zheng, H., & Finkelstein, D. (2009). Bayesian design using adult data to augment pediatric trials. *Clinical Trials*, 6(4): 297–304.

Sereni, F., Morselli, P., & Garattini, S. (1975). *Basic and Therapeutic Aspects of Perinatal Pharmacology. Monographs of the Mario Negri Institute for Pharmacological Research*. New York: Raven Press.

Spiegelhalter, D. J., Abrams, K. R., & Myles, J. P. (2004). *Bayesian Approaches to Clinical Trials and Health-Care Evaluation*. Chichester: John Wiley & Sons, Ltd.

Turner, S., Longworth, A., Nunn, A. J., & Choonara, I. (1998). Unlicensed and off label drug use in paediatric wards: Prospective study. *British Medical Journal*, 316(7128):343.

US Food and Drug Administration (FDA). (2014). *Draft Guidance for Industry: General Clinical Pharmacology Considerations for Pediatric Studies for Drugs and Biological Products*. Retrieved from http://www.fda.gov/downloads/Drugs/GuidanceComplianceRegulatoryInformation/Guidances/UCM425885.pdf

US Food and Drug Administration (FDA). (2016). *Leveraging Existing Clinical Data for Extrapolation to Pediatric Uses of Medical Devices*. Retrieved from https://www.fda.gov/media/91889/download

US Food and Drug Administration (FDA), & European Medicines Agency (EMA). (2021). *Common Commentary - EMA/FDA: Common Issues Requested for Discussion by the Respective Agency (EMA/PDCO and FDA) Concerning Paediatric Oncology Development Plans (Paediatric Investigation Plans [PIPs] and initial Pediatric Study Plans [iPSPs])*. Retrieved from https://www.ema.europa.eu/en/documents/other/common-commentary-ema/fda-common-issues-requested-discussion-respective-agency-ema/pdco-fda-concerning-paediatric-oncology-development-plans-paediatric-investigation-plans-pips_en.pdf

US Food and Drug Administration (FDA). (2005). *Guidance for Industry: How to Comply with the Pediatric Research Equity Act (PREA)*. Retrieved from https://www.fda.gov/media/72274/download

US Food and Drug Administration (FDA). (2017). *Pediatric Rare Diseases—A Collaborative Approach for Drug Development Using Gaucher Disease as a Model; Draft Guidance for Industry*. Retrieved from https://www.fda.gov/media/109465/download

US Food and Drug Administration (FDA). (2018a). *E11(R1) Addendum: Clinical Investigation of Medicinal Products in the Pediatric Population*. Retrieved from https://www.fda.gov/media/101398/download

US Food and Drug Administration (FDA). (2018b). *The History of Drug Regulation*. Retrieved from https://www.fda.gov/about-fda/fda-history/history-drug-regulation

US Food and Drug Administration (FDA). (2019a). *Accelerating Drug Development for Polyarticular Juvenile Idiopathic Arthritis (pJIA)*. Retrieved from https://www.fda.gov/news-events/fda-meetings-conferences-and-workshops/accelerating-drug-development-polyarticular-juvenile-idiopathic-arthritis-pjia-10022019-10022019

US Food and Drug Administration (FDA). (2019b). *Adaptive Design Clinical Trials for Drugs and Biologics Guidance for Industry*. Retrieved from https://www.fda.gov/media/78495/download

US Food and Drug Administration (FDA). (2019c). *Considerations for the Inclusion of Adolescent Patients in Adult Oncology Clinical Trials*. Retrieved from https://www.fda.gov/media/113499/download

US Food and Drug Administration (FDA). (2019d). *Enrichment Strategies for Clinical Trials to Support Approval of Human Drugs and Biological Products*. Retrieved from https://www.fda.gov/media/121320/download

US Food and Drug Administration (FDA). (2019e). *FDARA Implementation Guidance for Pediatric Studies of Molecularly Targeted Oncology Drugs: Amendments to Sec. 5050B of the FD&C Act*. Retrieved from https://www.fda.gov/media/133440/download

US Food and Drug Administration (FDA). (2019f). *General Clinical Pharmacology Considerations for Neonatal Studies for Drugs and Biological Products Guidance for Industry*. Retrieved from https://www.fda.gov/media/129532/download

US Food and Drug Administration (FDA). (2019g). *Guidance for Industry: Drugs for treatment of partial onset Seizures: Full Extrapolation of Efficacy from Adults to Pediatric Patients 2 Years of Age and Older*. Retrieved from https://www.fda.gov/media/130449/download

US Food and Drug Administration (FDA). (2019h). *Guidance for Industry: Severely Debilitating or Life-Threatening Hematologic Disorders: Nonclinical Development of Pharmaceuticals*. Retrieved from https://www.fda.gov/media/112750/download

US Food and Drug Administration (FDA). (2019i). *Patient-Focused Drug Development: Methods to Identify What Is Important to Patients. Draft Guidance*. Retrieved from https://www.fda.gov/media/131230/download

US Food and Drug Administration (FDA). (2019j). *Rare Diseases: Common Issues in Drug Development Guidance for Industry*. Retrieved from https://www.fda.gov/media/119757/download

US Food and Drug Administration (FDA). (2019k). *Rare Diseases: Natural History Studies for Drug Development Guidance for Industry. Draft Guidance*. Retrieved from https://www.fda.gov/media/122425/download

US Food and Drug Administration (FDA). (2019l). *Rare Pediatric Disease Priority Review Voucher*. Retrieved from https://www.fda.gov/media/90014/download

US Food and Drug Administration (FDA). (2020a). *Draft Guidance for Industry: Nonclinical Safety Evaluation of the Immunotoxic Potential of Drugs and Biologics*. Retrieved from https://www.fda.gov/media/135312/download

US Food and Drug Administration (FDA). (2020b). *International Collaboration/Pediatric Cluster*. Retrieved from https://www.fda.gov/science-research/pediatrics/international-collaboration-pediatric-cluster

US Food and Drug Administration (FDA). (2020c). *Patient-Focused Drug Development: Collecting Comprehensive and Representative Input Guidance for Industry, Food and Drug Administration Staff, and Other Stakeholders.* Retrieved from https://www.fda.gov/media/139088/download

US Food and Drug Administration (FDA). (2020d). *Pediatric Oncology Product Development Early Advice Meeting (Type F).* Retrieved from https://www.fda.gov/about-fda/oncology-center-excellence/pediatric-oncology-product-development-early-advice-meeting-type-f1

US Food and Drug Administration (FDA). (n.d.-a). *PDUFA Reauthorization Performance Goals and Procedures Fiscal Years 2018–2022.* Retrieved from https://www.fda.gov/media/99140/download. Accessed October 19, 2021.

US Food and Drug Administration (FDA). (n.d.-b). Retrieved from https://www.fda.gov/patients/learn-about-fda-patient-engagement

Viele, K., Berry, S., Neuenschwander, B., Amzal, B., Chen, F., Enas, N., ... & Thompson, L. (2014). Use of historical control data for assessing treatment effects in clinical trials. *Pharmaceutical Statistics,* 13(1): 41–54.

Wadsworth, I., Hampson, L. V., & Jaki, T. (2018). Extrapolation of efficacy and other data to support the development of new medicines for children: A systematic review of methods. *Statistical Methods in Medical Research,* 27(2): 398–413.

Wang, Y., Zhu, H., Madabushi, R., Liu, Q., Huang, S., & Zineh, I. (2019). Model-informed drug development: Current US regulatory practice and future considerations. *Clinical Pharmacology and Therapeutics.* https://doi.org/10.1002/cpt.1363.

Weber, K., Hemmings, R., & Koch, A. (2018). How to use prior knowledge and still give new data a chance? *Pharmaceutical Statistics,* 17: 329–341.

Wiesenfarth, M., & Calderazzo, S. (2020). Quantification of prior impact in terms of effective current sample size. *Biometrics,* 76: 326–336.

Woodcock, J., & LaVange, L. M. (2017). Master protocols to study multiple therapies, multiple diseases, or both. *New England Journal of Medicine,* 377: 62–70. https://doi.org/10.1056/NEJMra1510062.

Ye, J., Reaman, G., De Claro, R., & Sridhara, R. (2020). A Bayesian approach in design and analysis of pediatric cancer clinical trials. *Pharmaceutical Statistics,* 19(6): 814–826.

Zhu, H., Huang, S., Madabushi, R., Strauss, D. G., Wang, Y., & Zineh, I. (2019). Model-informed drug development: A regulatory perspective on progress. *Clinical Pharmacology and Therapeutics.* https://doi.org/10.1002/cpt.1475.

Notes

1 https://www.ema.europa.eu/en/partners-networks/patients-consumers#framework-for-interaction-section
2 Revised framework for interaction between the European Medicines Agency and patients and consumers and their organizations European Medicines Agency. October 2014.
3 https://www.fda.gov/media/154449/download

7

Use of Modeling and Simulation in Support of Drug Development for Rare Diseases

Mark Peterson and Brenda Cirincione

Vertex Pharmaceuticals

CONTENTS

7.1 Introduction to Modeling and Simulation in Rare Diseases

An overriding challenge in the clinical development of novel therapeutics for rare diseases is aptly captured in the first word of the descriptor – rare. Rarity is manifested in both the number of patients, as well as often the amount of information (often samples) that can be obtained from patients being treated, and from which we desire to quantify drug effects. In the face of limited data, data-analytic disciplines are looked to for generating information sufficient to assess a therapeutic candidate's potential benefit. To interpret the available data and support future trial designs, researchers employ sophisticated modeling and simulation methodologies, construct plausible mathematical expressions to describe observations, and leverage the data that they have. Often, these methods fit data collected across time, studies, compound types, patient characteristics, treatment statuses, and even sometimes across diseases. The models are often structured in ways that allow estimation of data central tendencies, as well as distributions to create probabilistic predictions similar to weather forecasts that state the possibility of rain or snow. In doing so, they allow us to draw inference about the generalizability of observations, build confidence in our understanding, and provide predictive platforms to answer design and relationship questions, thereby supporting therapeutic advancement. In this chapter, the reader will be provided a glimpse of how and why modeling of data from within a patient over time, and across patients – more formally referred to as repeated-measures mixed-effects modeling – is used to generate these inferences and evidence to support drug development decisions, particularly in the rare disease setting. The aim is to provide the reader a practical "context of use" view of the most common types of pharmaceutically applied model classes and how they commonly are used and potentially may be extended in future to help scientists assess treatments for rare diseases.

While many methods are available to scientists for fitting mathematical expressions to data, over the last quarter century, the global drug development community has formally recognized the discipline of predictive modeling and simulation with repeated-measures (often time series) mixed-effects methods in clinical drug development as pharmacometrics (PMx). One well-established definition of PMx is "The science of developing and applying mathematical and statistical methods to characterize, understand, and predict a drug's pharmacokinetic, pharmacodynamic, and biomarker outcome behavior" [1]. PMx is also the underpinning scientific discipline utilized in the globally recognized drug development approach referred to as model-informed drug development (MIDD). "One definition of MIDD is an approach that involves developing and applying exposure-based, biological and statistical models derived from preclinical and clinical data sources to inform drug development and decision- making. It aims to integrate information from diverse data sources to help decrease uncertainty and lower failure rates, and to develop information that cannot or would not be generated experimentally" [2].

Collectively, they define the industry understanding of certain classes of modeling methods applied in pharmaceutical development (i.e., PMx) as being implemented according to a paradigm aimed at generating statistics supporting drug development decisions (MIDD). Currently, MIDD is recognized by industry and regulatory agencies as the structural paradigm by which PMx can be critically evaluated and leveraged to facilitate development and review of therapies, and notably for orphan/rare diseases. In an effort to harmonize and provide efficiencies for the ways in which MIDD is executed, the International Council for Harmonisation of Technical Requirements for Pharmaceuticals for Human Use (ICH), a global committee that provides pharmaceutical guidelines, recently endorsed a plan to develop an overarching guidance addressing many principles and practices associated with MIDD activities and outputs [3]. This effort has the potential to move the global community closer to having a unified approach to supporting the use of PMx in the generation of evidence for vetting treatments, including those for rare diseases. Therefore, the application of PMx and integration of MIDD principles into the development of therapies for rare diseases, where data paucity is a reality, is supported by global regulatory institutions and provides a method for integrating and maximally leveraging available data in the assessment of therapeutic candidates.

In this chapter, we provide a practical description of the major model classes followed by some applications of modeling and simulation in rare diseases. The chapter is divided into four sections. The first section is the introduction you are reading now. That is followed by a section on the most common methodological classes of PMx models that underpin modeling and simulation's ability to leverage data for rare diseases. Next, examples of those modeling and simulation classes in rare diseases are presented, with their benefits to the drug development process highlighted. And lastly, an aspirational view of future potentials for applying modeling and simulation in rare diseases suggests some alternate means for bringing life-saving medications to patients suffering with rare diseases faster than current practices. Throughout, the reader is provided information from which to reflect on the challenges data paucity poses, the presented methodologies, and the potential benefits and opportunities for applied modeling and simulation in the rare disease domain of drug development.

7.2 Modeling Methodologies Suited to Rare Diseases

Through the lens of rare diseases, PMx methods can be seen as particularly valuable in their ability to be developed using sparse data collected across limited numbers of patients to generate inferences that complement traditional analyses. To accomplish this, PMx methods often use all the available time-series data collected in patients, from screening through follow-up, and including any specific timepoint of interest (e.g., a landmark timepoint of the primary endpoint). Doing so results in a model structure that is suitable for simulations that can expand the understanding of a drug candidate's potential. These simulations may include both interpolation and extrapolation in dimensions of interest. Commonly, simulated quantities include predictions of alternate drug exposures or effects, forecasts of events further out in time, examinations of distributional possibilities in larger or different populations, and more. To accomplish this, scientist can draw on an extensive number of computer programs, fitting minimization algorithms, and applied statistical methodologies – a breadth that is far beyond the remit of this text. Therefore, here we provide a brief, practical, explanation of some key aspects of PMx modeling principles and describe, at a high level, the most frequently encountered classes of modeling methods. After which, examples of these class uses are presented in the next section of the chapter, entitled "Applications to Rare Diseases". For a more thorough treatment of these topics and beyond, the reader may want to explore Gabrielsson and Weiner's Pharmacokinetic and Pharmacodynamic Data Analysis for model selection and structure information, and/or Ette and Williams' Pharmacometrics, The Science of Quantitative Pharmacology for methodologies and applications [1,4]. In short, a PMx model can be thought of as a related collection of mathematical expressions that appropriately represent the observed data, with multiple levels of variability estimated. Models that estimate multiple levels of variability are referred to as mixed-effects or multilevel models. A notable characteristic of PMx models is the routine invocation of nonlinear mathematical expressions in the models to describe the observed data. Therefore, when a PMx model is fit to data arising from multiple study subjects simultaneously, and multiple levels of variability are estimated, the full descriptor used is population nonlinear mixed-effects models.

There are three distinct layers (or levels) of parameters in many PMx models. The first core level in a PMx model is the math that describes the measurement(s) of interest as a function of time or some other independent variable. This math is referred to as the structural model and can take on any form necessary to describe the overall shape of the data. Commonly, a series of ordinary differential equations (ODEs) are linked by one equation using a quantity from another of the equations. There can be as many ODEs as necessary to describe the data and system giving rise to the data. At the same time, principals of parsimony are usually respected and only the number of expressions and parameters required to provide description of the observed data and a fit-for-purpose use are included and estimated. It is also worth noting that sometimes, these ODEs have explicit solutions, and those can be used to expedite the fitting process. And, in some cases, PMx models can be non-ODEs and simple mathematical expressions. Regardless of the structure, the main parameters of the mathematical expressions in a mixed-effects (or multilevel) model are called fixed effects as they are not estimates of distributions – simply point values. Next are parameters that describe how the fixed-effect parameters change from patient to patient. Those distributional parameters are often referred to as between-subject or intersubject variability. With fixed and between-subject variance terms included, the model can be estimated and provides individual specific fits, with a curve for each subject's data, and estimates of the variances in parameters. But, there is one level left to estimate, and that is residual variability. With the individual lines fitted through each subjects' data, there will be unexplained differences between the observed data and the fitted line. This can arise from multiple potential sources including but not limited to assay error, collection time error, and patient variability in clinical measures. Regardless of how it arises, the differences between the predicted points and the observed data can be estimated and described as a distribution of differences referred to as residual variability. Collectively, the PMx model provides a model structure that suitably captures the trajectory and distribution of the available data and can simulate new data using the estimates of fixed effects, random effects, and residual effects that arise from the observed data used in the model.

The most prominent class of PMx models used in clinical drug development is population pharmacokinetic and pharmacodynamic (popPK; popPKPD) models. These models employ mixed-effect paradigms as just described and quantify drug concentrations (PK) and measures of drug effects (PD) from a population of patients collected with full and/or sparse sampling strategies. They find use in advancing potential therapeutics by their ability to predict drug exposures at previously studied or alternate doses, forecast PK and/ or PD out in time, and estimate distributional and probabilistic outcomes. However, another extremely useful feature of PMx models is the ability to identify and incorporate predictor variables. In the context of PMx, predictors are more commonly called covariates and routinely enter models on between-subject variability terms. In doing so, they partition the variability in the observed data into explained (by the covariate) and unexplained between-subject variability. While their addition does not reduce the observed variability in PK or PD, it allows us to quantify the contribution to the variability from the covariates included. This is useful when it comes to understanding where variability arises from and for predicting alternate outcomes. At the same time, the way in which covariates enter the models can often represent meaningful physiologic associations, such as allometric relationships between weight and clearance–as often seen in pediatrics. Once informative covariates are established and checked, the full model can be used to evaluate various relevant aspects of clinical import via simulation, such as the joint impact of all the included covariates, their impact at the extremes, and other design elements. In all cases, adequate model evaluation and assumption checking, as described in many regulatory guidances, are conducted to ensure the model is fit for purpose for its intended use [5,6].

Two other model classes commonly used in clinical drug development that tend to be more complex than traditional popPK or popPKPD models are physiologically based pharmacokinetic (PBPK) and quantitative systems pharmacology (QSP) models. These two classes of models have found uses in clinical development and also can be applicable to the entire drug development life cycle. PBPK and QSP models could be considered exceptions to the parsimony approach, but there are benefits to the included complexities. Because of their structure and rationale in being built, they tend to mathematically represent the physiology involved in the drug's pharmacology. To be more specific, a PBPK model has mathematical expressions representing numerous regions and organs of the body that are of interest for the drug being developed. These compartments are usually informed via preclinical experiments or with knowledge iteratively developed through clinical investigation. Into this physiologic construct, elements of biology and physiology that are relevant to the drug effect are incorporated to allow for model fitting and simulation similar to those conducted with the popPK model. PBPK models can be extremely useful when there are questions about circulating concentrations, and we need to understand the distributional properties of a drug candidate. Therefore, while the multiple additional compartments are not necessarily directly supported by observed clinical data, their inclusion in the model provides inferences of import to the drug candidate in a way that would otherwise not be feasible to generate in clinical study. QSP models are like PBPK models in terms of increased mathematical complexity, yet differ in their perspective, linkages, and application. Both modeling approaches use systems of equations representing more fully (than PopPK) the underlying physiology of the human body. However, QSP models tend to be focused more on depicting the links between phenomena of physiology and/or endocrinology relevant to a specific drug or pharmacology, whereas PBPK is focused on the volume flows to the various tissues and organs of the body, reflecting the vascular system in their structure. This leads to QSP and PBPK models being similar in their degree of complexity as compared to popPK, but tending to be used in different ways due to their structure.

A model class that is a departure from models considering drug disposition is disease progression models. This class of models is aimed at describing in as simple as form as possible the clinical endpoint in the patient as it changes over the natural progression of the disease. Often, this is on the background of some active therapy, but maybe in the absence of any treatment whatsoever in the case of some rare diseases. Similar to the other classes of models described, disease progression models can be made up of a series of ODEs, or simply some time-dependent relationship that can describe the change in the clinical endpoint over time. As with popPKPD, disease progression is often described by repeated-measures mixed-effects models. In rare diseases, because there is a limitation in the patient pool, natural history data, registry data, and placebo arms from prior executed randomized control trials provide valuable data to the quantification of disease progression. Therefore, PMx modeling methods have a unique opportunity to utilize the totality of data collected to bring understanding and inference to what is expected to occur in patients in the absence of therapeutic intervention.

In the end, all of the classes of models that exist for use in drug development have the same paradigm for use – they must describe, as well as possible, the observed data. They must be able to (1) return that data via simulation (in-sample reliability); (2) provide simulated outcomes that are realistic, and (3) respect the natural limits of the observed data (out-of-sample reliability).

7.3 Application to Rare Diseases

The ability of PMx repeated-measures mixed-effects models to leverage data in rare diseases has been realized in numerous ways and is consistent with the general trend that is visible in the number of filings between 2000 and 2015 that contain documented use of modeling (Figure 7.1). Of the 192 filings that documented the use of modeling in them, the majority were PK and PopPK modeling, followed by exposure response (ER) and PD, PBPK, and QSP modeling (Figure 7.2).

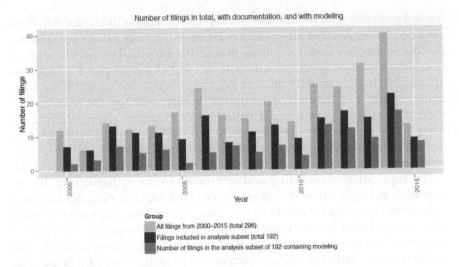

FIGURE 7.1
Number of filings in total, with documentation, and with modeling from 2000 to 2015 [7].

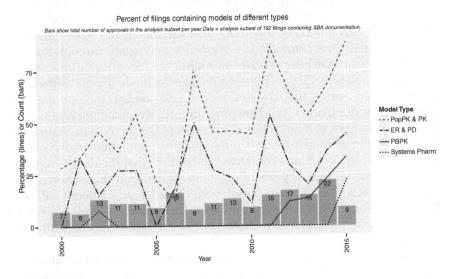

FIGURE 7.2
Percent of filings containing models of different types [7].

In some cases, the ability to use models, based upon understood physiology, biology, and rational assumptions, to draw inferences in the face of data paucity is often critical to addressing drug development challenges. In principle, the biggest challenge in rare and orphan diseases is overcoming the data paucity that derives from the small populations of patients. A resulting tradeoff becomes deriving as much information as possible from limited available data versus extension of trial execution timelines. But, there are also challenges that are readily overcome in robust patient populations that become nearly insurmountable in rare disease populations. The application of quantitative approaches as outlined in PUDFA VI provide tools and approaches to data scarcity that can help to integrate and quantify the areas of uncertainty that naturally arise in rare diseases [8]. Over the past 20 years, industry has generated a broad collection of examples demonstrating the ways modeling and simulation can inform decisions in all types of drug development, including rare diseases. The advancement of models from simplistic empirical models to advance mechanistic models has been applied [9].

The application of modeling and simulation in the pediatric rare disease area is an example where the integration of the totality of evidence is critical to facilitate bringing treatment to the youngest patients. The notion of pediatric extrapolation is even more critical in the rare disease space where the number of patients is even smaller. FDA pediatric guidance specifically calls out that extrapolation of efficacy from adults to pediatrics might be possible based on three conditions, similar disease process, similar response to therapy, and the same indication as those studied in older patients [10]. One of the examples of the use of extrapolation to bring therapies to pediatrics patients with rare diseases is with cystic fibrosis. Throughout the development of therapies for cystic fibrosis, modeling and simulation has been employed to empower pediatric extrapolation of efficacy and safety through the process of exposure matching [11–14]. As highlighted in a recent manuscript on Trikafta results in CF patients aged 6–11 years, modeling and simulation was integrated during the trial to establish and confirm the optimal dose in this patient population [15]. This program utilized modeling and simulation-based analyses of data collected in Part A of the protocol to confirm the planned dosing scheme for Part B. Subsequently, population analysis of the data collected in Part B was conducted to confirm that the dosing regimen exposure achieved in 6–11 years of age subjects matched those shown to be safe and efficacious in ≥12 years population. These PK simulations confirmed the optimal weight cutoff for the transition between dose levels of Trikafta for this age-group. Similar approaches have been reported across other CF therapies [15–18].

While data paucity is an overarching challenge, the generation of certain types of data adds additional hurdles to addressing otherwise routine regulatory concerns. Several elements of trial design and a drug label where this is notable are in the clinical starting dose and drug interactions and specific populations label sections, respectively. Fortunately, PBPK models and in-silico tools for predicting metabolic pathways for compounds based on substituent groups and chemical structure have gained increasing acceptance over the years [19]. While they do not provide a complete substitute for in vitro experiments, and in some cases the need for clinical trials, they can provide important inference. As highlighted above, PBPK is a mechanistic modeling approach that can help with determination of likely changes in required doses for special populations and in difficult to study situations [20]. Studying the need for dose adjustments in rare diseases is difficult, and in some cases not feasible. This application of PBPK in rare diseases is growing. The examples of the use include informing the dosing regimens for hydrocortisone replacement for children and adults with cortisol deficiency [21]. The analyses presented describe a robust approach of PBPK modeling and subsequent simulations for hydrocortisone to provide dosing recommendations for a modified release formulation for a pediatric population [21]. Rioux and Waters authored a mini-review in 2016 where they reviewed the use of PBPK in oncology drug development as well as PBPK model use in "a prospective manner to inform the first pediatric trials of pinometostat and tazemetostat in genetically defined populations" [22]. They compiled a table of PBPK modeling applications within pediatric oncology drug development (Table 7.1) and note that most commonly, pediatric PBPK modeling is accomplished by scaling a validated adult PBPK model to children by incorporating ontogeny and maturation processes, thereby avoiding preclinical-to-clinical interspecies scaling and differences. Importantly, the table describes the objectives of the PBPK modeling and the software used to conduct the analyses. While most of the examples were not performed prior to the first in patient studies, the last three cases point out the ability to use these methods to inform trial decisions a priori.

QSP models represent another class of models that have emerged in drug development over the past two decades. They have gained visibility as tools capable of generating useful inferences about therapeutic mechanisms and likely clinical outcomes by joint fitting of multiple disease data sources simultaneously. These data sources are often at scales from cellular mechanisms up to clinical outcomes. Through the construction of in silico physiology, the fitting of the multiple data sources at various scales enables the QSP model's ability to accommodate nonlinearities in phenomena and feedback mechanisms. Importantly, since they are built to represent the physiology and disease of interest in a fit-for-purpose way, they hold the potential to bridge gaps in data quantity in the rare disease space. Therefore, the tradeoff of added complexity compared to traditional popPKPD models for increased inference can in some cases add significant value for forecasting a therapeutic's potential. The following case provides recent examples of QSP models in the rare disease acid sphingomyelinase deficiency (ASMD).

Sometimes, PBPK models are integrated into QSP models to provide both a dispositional representation of the therapeutic and a description of the mechanistic basis for its effects. A recent example was provided by Kaddi et al. in their publication of QSP modeling of ASMD and treatment with the enzyme replacement therapy (ERT) olipudase alfa [23]. ASMD, commonly known as Niemann—Pick disease type A and B, is a rare disease, effects both men and women with a prevalence estimated to be 1 in 250,000 in the general population, and is both serious and potentially fatal. The causality is mutations in the SMPD1 gene which encodes ASM. In the absence of ASM, sphingomyelin, a major constituent of cell membranes, is not metabolized to ceramide. This

TABLE 7.1

Summary of PBPK Modeling Applications in Pediatric Oncology Drug Development [22]

Drug	Route of Administration	Objective(s)	Software	Data Used in Model Build	Performed Prior to FTP[a]	Reference
Busulfan	i.v.	Predict plasma concentration–time curves	PK-Sim (Bayer Technology Services, Germany)	Adult	No	Diestelhorst et al. (2014)
Cisplatin	i.v.	Describe the PBPK model development; simulate cisplatin disposition in humans	Not reported	Dog	No	Evans et al. (1982)
Docetaxel	i.v.	Demonstrate how PBPK modeling can be applied to optimize dose and sampling times for a pediatric PK bridging study in oncology	Simcyp (Certara, UK)	Adult	No	Thai et al. (2015)
Etoposide	i.v.	Evaluate the ability of PBPK to predict the systemic drug exposure in children and the effect of comedications	PK-Sim	Adult	No	Kersting et al. (2012)
Imatinib	p.o.	Predict plasma concentration–time profiles in plasma and tissue in pediatric subjects and assess the effect of pediatric growth processes using a PBPK model. Evaluate factors influencing imatinib exposure in pediatric patients	Not reported	Adult	No	European Medicines Agency (2013)
6-Mercaptopurine	i.v. and p.o.	Improve dose individualization and dosage regimen optimization; model DDI interaction with methotrexate	MATLAB (Mathworks, Natick, MA)	Adult	No	Ogungbenro et al. (2014b)

(Continued)

TABLE 7.1 (Continued)

Summary of PBPK Modeling Applications in Pediatric Oncology Drug Development [22]

Drug	Route of Administration	Objective(s)	Software	Data Used in Model Build	Performed Prior to FTP[a]	Reference
Methotrexate	i.v. and p.o.	Evaluate the role of modeling and simulation in the development of drugs for rare diseases	MATLAB	Adult	No	Ogungbenro et al. (2014a)
Methotrexate	i.v.	Evaluate the effect of malignant effusions on the PK of methotrexate	Berkeley Madonna (University of California–Berkeley, Berkeley, CA)	Adult	No	Li and Gwilt (2002)
Obatoclax	i.v.	Evaluate the potential to achieve target exposures in infants	PK-Sim	Mouse	Yes	Barrett et al. (2011)
Pinometostat	i.v.	First time in pediatrics starting dose selection	Simcyp	Adult	Yes	Waters et al. (2014)
Tazemetostat	p.o.	First time in pediatrics starting dose selection	GastroPlus (Simulations Plus, Lancaster, CA)	Adult	Yes	Rioux et al. (2015)

[a] First time in pediatrics.

results in its intracellular accumulation in multiple organs and manifestations such as hepatosplenomegaly, infiltrative lung disease, hematological abnormalities, and dyslipidemia, which produce a range of visceral and neurovisceral disease subtypes. The most severe of these subtypes, infantile neurovisceral (Niemann–Pick type A), is fatal with patients typically succumbing by age 3. The aim of developing the QSP model was to provide a model construct that was able to describe the multiple clinical endpoints and PD measures of import in ASMD simultaneously with one construct and to use the model to begin to understand the mechanistic reasons for patient variability. To accomplish this, the authors developed the model requiring it to describe in vitro cell line data, data from preclinical studies in knockout mice, from natural history studies, and from ongoing clinical trials with ERT. It consisted of four sub-models: (1) a molecular level model; (2) a cellular level model; (3) an organ level model; and (4) a reduced PBPK model focusing on three organ compartments of interest. The PBPK model was reduced from its original published form as a fit-for-purpose adaptation, while still retaining the flow characteristics for the organs of import. Unique to PBPK and QSP, the various sources of data can be used to inform the interplay between the organs, cells, and drug disposition and aid in the overall estimation of the model parameters as shown in Table 7.2.

Once built, the QSP model was validated and used to support further development of ASMD treatment with olipudase alfa in progressively younger patients. The model enables the evaluation of disease and response similarities and differences across the disease sub-types and in populations of differing ages, hence differing PK. It provides a platform to evaluate multiple endpoints and PD markers simultaneously, thereby increasing the confidence in the extrapolations. The model also serves as a structure from which hypotheses about the disease sub-types can be tested for plausibility. This is accomplished uniquely in QSP models because the parameters have specific attributes and associations with body regions in the case of the PBPK

TABLE 7.2

Overview of Data Sources Used to Develop and Calibrate the ASMD QSP Model [23]

Data Source	Model Level	Description
Preclinical studies (ASMKO mouse) [22]	PBPK	Estimation of PK and biodistribution parameters from ASMKO PBPK model, which were then scaled to human PBPK model
Natural history study (59 adult and pediatric patients, from 1 year to up to 11 years of assessment) [20]	Organ	Estimation of disease progression rates in lungs and spleen
Phase Ia (11 adult patients) [21]	PBPK	Dose response and calibration of human PK model
Phase Ib (five adult patients) [8]	PBPK, molecular, organ	Calibration of endpoints in molecular-level and organ-level models

components and mechanisms in the case of the cellular components. Then, the manifestations of such changes can be explored by evaluation of the organ level and clinical outcomes that arise. Therefore, the ASMD QSP model has the potential to provide in silico treatment assessment of pediatrics and disease sub-types in advance of clinical trials, thereby informing the design and increasing confidence in the outcome. It also provides a foundation from which other therapeutic's mechanisms and disposition can be incorporated and used in comparative assessments made of drug efficacy. Particularly in rare diseases, such inference from QSP models to inform drug development advancement decisions and/or selection of candidates for advancement prior to time-consuming and costly execution of clinical trials is useful.

In the area of gene and cell therapies, there is no drug concentration per se, and applications of PMx are emerging that use natural history data to understand disease progression in patients. The aim of modeling in these settings is to develop understanding of the changes that would be anticipated to occur in patient endpoints in the absence of treatment and the predictors (i.e., covariates) that should be considered as contributing to variability in disease trajectory. Once the influential predictors are quantified via modeling, they can become elements of trial design inclusion/exclusion criteria as a means of providing a more homogeneous patient population.

Recently, this approach has been applied in Duchenne muscular dystrophy (DMD) [24]. To understand the dynamics of change and sources of variability in five clinical endpoints, the Duchenne Regulatory Science Consortium (D-RSC) in collaboration with the Critical Path Institute (CPath) and others integrated data from 15 natural history studies, registries, and placebo arms of randomized controlled studies in DMD patients into a single standardized and quality controlled analysis dataset of 1,505 patients with 27,252 observations. The dataset was assembled according to the regulatory acceptable format, structure, and terminology defined for Clinical Data Interchange Standards Consortium (CDISC) standard in DMD [25]. Using this broad, unified dataset, repeated-measures, mixed-effects models were developed that described the dynamics of change of each of the five endpoints (velocities of time to stand from supine, time to climb four stairs, 10-m walk/run time, Northstar Ambulatory Assessment, and forced vital capacity). Because of the nature of the dataset, the evaluation of predictors was limited to variables that are most commonly collected and of interest to clinical researchers — steroid treatment, genetic mutation, race, weight, height, and baseline function. However, collectively, these predictors accounted for approximately 50% of the observed variance in the population. The result of this effort was a web-based clinical trial simulation tool that can be used to simulate plausible future outcomes under varying baseline patient conditions and characteristics, based on the totality of data and represented by the model structures. The tool is able to generate the uncertainty and most likely outcome for any of the five clinical endpoints conditional on criteria the user selects, such as the magnitude of anticipated drug effect, the range of the demographic characteristics, the cohort size, and the duration of an intended study. This process can be repeated and the simulated results for an endpoint of interest under different criteria explored and compared. An example of such output was provided in a poster at World Muscle Society 2020 conference, and the intent is to make these simulation platforms publicly available once regulatory endorsement from both FDA and EMA is obtained [26].

7.4 Future Opportunities for Modeling in Rare Diseases

As drug development aims to deliver treatments for increasingly rare diseases, the demands on methods used to analyze data and convert it into decision-making information will also increase. As has been described, many of the repeated-measures mixed-effect modeling methods available today were developed to utilize sparse data and provide inference about the distributions giving rise to that data. In the future, we will need to do more with even less. We will need to be able to draw understanding not only from sparse sampling but also under conditions of sparse populations. The result will be a reduction in the information content available to the researcher from which to make decisions. This will put even greater pressure on our methodologies and data sources, as well as how we use both to understand these increasingly rare diseases.

From the methodological perspective, data analytic tools and approaches to estimating data trends, data central tendencies, and data variance in PK and/ or PD continue to evolve. While NONMEM is still considered the gold standard by many regulatory agencies today, alternate computational platforms have emerged in the last couple decades. While similar in their ability to support the conduct of complex multilevel/mixed-effects modeling, these newer platforms are built on modern programming languages with an aim toward being faster and supportive of more complex computation. Additionally, the computational power available to scientists is enabling Bayesian algorithms and analysis options to become more prevalent and provide further statistically applicable options for analysis of sparse data. Together, the tools at the disposal of scientists to conduct complex analyses of both endpoints and longitudinal observations, infer variability, describe disease progression, and forecast future observations will continue to advance. The use of advances in pharmacostatistical methodologies and tools will become increasingly critical to developing therapies for rare diseases as data availability becomes more limited.

From the regulatory perspective, processes and regulations governing methods and data use will continue to evolve in ways that enable maximal understanding from limited data. Presently, several regulatory efforts are aimed at how models are used to support knowledge generation in the evaluation of novel therapies. The effort mentioned previously being undertaken by ICH MIDD working group to establish unified approaches to the application of model informed drug development principles on a global level is aimed at reducing differences in expectations for model use across the international regulatory bodies. The objective is to harmonize worldwide, as much as possible, how modeling work is reported, qualified, and methodologically executed. It is also reasonable to believe that in the future, the trickier questions of adequate evidence derived from modeling to support a drug approval maybe a topic of discussion within ICH. The challenge of generating adequate evidence under conditions of limited information content as in rare diseases has gained visibility within the United States via the FDA complex innovative design and model informed drug development pilot programs. These programs aim to engage drug development sponsors and regulatory stakeholders in conversations to align in advance on trial designs and methodological plans to generate evidence supporting novel therapy approval. The overall intent is to provide adequate evidence of efficacy and safety with less patient burden where possible and still meet the regulatory expectations for doing so. Lastly, as described in Chapter 5, regulations regarding the use of real-world data outline criteria and conditions under which natural history data may be considered for use to support demonstration of efficacy and safety. This is particularly important to the rare disease area where data are sparse and such data can provide a means to build understanding of disease progression. The construction of disease progression models with rare disease data is one important avenue for sparing patients from placebo treatments and hastens trial completions in the future. Together, the emergence of faster, diverse, well-established pharmacostatistical methods and regulations supporting their use, along with the use of real-world data, suggests a promising paradigm that is beginning to be realized [27].

In conclusion, current and emerging efforts to use modeling and simulation in rare diseases constitute an investment of time and resources in charting a path toward the use of existing data and models more systematically and systemically for the generation of quantitative evidence of a therapeutics potential. As we move forward, our ability to leverage existing information using advanced analytical modeling methods to generate more understanding and evidence with less data will have direct implications on patients and our ability to support drug approvals in rare diseases in the future. And while there is a natural lower limit to how much data one needs to generate solid inference, there are still opportunities to improve upon our current practices for the welfare of patients suffering with rare diseases.

References

1. Ette, E.I. and P.J. Williams, *Pharmacometrics: The Science of Quantitative Pharmacology*. 2007, Hoboken, NJ: Wiley; Chichester: John Wiley [distributor].
2. FDA.gov. *CDER Conversation: Model Informed Drug Development*. [URL] 2018 06/12/2018; Raj Madabushi, Ph.D., Team Leader, Guidance and Policy Team, Office of Translational Sciences, Office of Clinical Pharmacology, CDER]. Available from: https://www.fda.gov/drugs/news-events-human-drugs/cder-conversation-model-informed-drug-development.

3. ICH. *Press Release: ICH Assembly Virtual Meeting, November 2021*. 2021 [cited 2021 25 November 2021]; New areas of ICH harmonisation]. Available from: https://www.ich.org/pressrelease/press-release-ich-assembly-virtual-meeting-november-2021.

4. Gabrielsson, J. and D. Weiner, *Pharmacokinetic—Pharmacodynamic Data Analysis: Concepts and Applications*. 2nd ed. 1997, Stockholm, Sweden: Apotekarsocieteten, p. 770.

5. EMEA. *Guideline on Reporting the Results of Population Pharmacokinetic Analyses*. [pdf] 2007 21 June 2007; European Regulatory Guidance]. Available from: https://www.ema.europa.eu/en/documents/scientific-guideline/guideline-reporting-results-population-pharmacokinetic-analyses_en.pdf.

6. FDA, *Population Pharmacokinetics Guidance for Industry*, C.f.D.E.a. Research and C.f.B.E.a. Research, Editors. 2022, FDA: https://www.fda.gov/media/128793/download.

7. Gastonguay. *Modeling & Simulation: Filling the Knowledge Gap in Rare Diseases*. Return on Investment on the Utilization of Systems Pharmacology and Pharmacometrics in Drug Development for Rare Diseases: Challenges and Opportunities [Presentation] 2015 September 26, 2015; ACCP Workshop]. Figures developed by Janelle Hajjar Lenie, PhD. Available from: https://www.metrumrg.com/wp-content/uploads/2015/09/Gastonguay_ACCP_2015.pdf.

8. FDA. *PDUFA VI: Fiscal Years 2018–2022*. Prescription Drug User Fee Amendments 2018 07/07/2020 [cited 2021 01/21/2022]; Available from: https://www.fda.gov/industry/prescription-drug-user-fee-amendments/pdufa-vi-fiscal-years-2018-2022.

9. Wang, Y. and S.M. Huang, Commentary on fit-for-purpose models for regulatory applications. *J Pharm Sci*, 2019. **108**(1): pp. 18–20.

10. United States Department of Health and Human Services. Food and Drug Administration. Center for Drug Evaluation and Research (CDER), Center for Biologics Evaluation and Research (CBER). *Guidance for Industry E11 Clinical Investigation of Medicinal Products in the Pediatric Population*. 2000.

11. European Medicines Agency., *Reflection paper on the use of extrapolation in the development of medicines for paediatrics*. 2018.

12. United States Department of Health and Human Services. Food and Drug Administration. Center for Drug Evaluation and Research (CDER), *General Clinical Pharmacology Considerations for Pediatric Studies for Drugs and Biological Products Guidance for Industry*, C.f.D.E.a.R. (CDER), Editor. 2014.

13. Mulugeta, Y., et al., Exposure matching for extrapolation of efficacy in pediatric drug development. *J Clin Pharmacol*, 2016. **56**(11): pp. 1326–1334.

14. Dunne, J., et al., Extrapolation of adult data and other data in pediatric drug-development programs. *Pediatrics*, 2011. **128**(5): pp. e1242–e1249.

15. Zemanick, E.T., et al., A phase 3 open-label study of elexacaftor/tezacaftor/ivacaftor in children 6 through 11 years of age with cystic fibrosis and at least one F508del allele. *Am J Respir Crit Care Med*, 2021. **203**(12): pp. 1522–1532.

16. Davies, J.C., et al., Safety, pharmacokinetics, and pharmacodynamics of ivacaftor in patients aged 2–5 years with cystic fibrosis and a CFTR gating mutation (KIWI): an open-label, single-arm study. *Lancet Respir Med*, 2016. **4**(2): pp. 107–115.

17. Davies, J.C., et al., Ivacaftor in infants aged 4 to <12 months with cystic fibrosis and a gating mutation. Results of a two-part phase 3 clinical trial. *Am J Respir Crit Care Med*, 2021. **203**(5): pp. 585–593.

18. McNamara, J.J., et al., Safety, pharmacokinetics, and pharmacodynamics of lumacaftor and ivacaftor combination therapy in children aged 2–5 years with cystic fibrosis homozygous for F508del-CFTR: an open-label phase 3 study. *Lancet Respir Med*, 2019. **7**(4): pp. 325–335.

19. Grimstein, M., et al., Physiologically based pharmacokinetic modeling in regulatory science: an update from the U.S. Food and Drug Administration's Office of Clinical Pharmacology. *J Pharm Sci*, 2019. **108**(1): pp. 21–25.

20. Howard, M., et al., Dose adjustment in orphan disease populations: the quest to fulfill the requirements of physiologically based pharmacokinetics. *Expert Opin Drug Metab Toxicol*, 2018. **14**(12): pp. 1315–1330.

21. Bonner, J.J., et al., Development and verification of an endogenous PBPK model to inform hydrocortisone replacement dosing in children and adults with cortisol deficiency. *Eur J Pharm Sci*, 2021. **165**: pp. 105913.

22. Rioux, N. and N.J. Waters, Physiologically based pharmacokinetic modeling in pediatric oncology drug development. *Drug Metab Dispos*, 2016. **44**(7): pp. 934–43.

23. Kaddi, C.D., et al., Quantitative systems pharmacology modeling of acid sphingomyelinase deficiency and the enzyme replacement therapy olipudase alfa is an innovative tool for linking pathophysiology and pharmacology. *CPT Pharmacometrics Syst Pharmacol*, 2018. **7**(7): pp. 442–452.

24. Lingineni, K., et al., Development of a model-based clinical trial simulation platform to optimize the design of clinical trials for Duchenne muscular dystrophy. *CPT Pharmacometrics Syst Pharmacol*, 2021. **11**(3): pp. 318–332.

25. CDISC. *Duchenne Muscular Dystrophy Therapeutic Area User Guide v1.0. 2017* [cited 25 September 2017]; Available from: https://www.cdisc.org/standards/therapeutic-areas/duchenne-muscular-dystrophy.

26. Berg, A., *Development of a regulatory-ready clinical trial simulation tool for Duchenne muscular dystrophy - Jane Larkindale - , Sarah Kim*, 2021. Critical Path Institute. Available from: https://policycommons.net/artifacts/1730699/development-of-a-regulatory-ready-clinical-trial-simulation-tool-for-duchenne-muscular-dystrophy/2462348/.

27. Jahanshahi, M., et al., The use of external controls in FDA regulatory decision making. *Ther Innov Regul Sci*, 2021. **55**(5): pp. 1019–1035.

8

Case Studies of Rare Disease Drug Development

CONTENTS

8.1 Use of Natural History Studies for Drug Approval: A Case Study of Zolgensma® (Onasemnogene Abeparvovec-Xioi)

Yimeng Lu
Vir Biotechnology

Chenkun Wang
Vertex Pharmaceuticals

8.1.1 Background

Cell and gene therapy (CGT), one of the new frontiers in pharmaceutical industry, is experiencing rapid growth in recent years due to significant scientific advancements and the clinical promise of these new innovations. By 2025, it is anticipated that the FDA will approve 10–20 CGT products a year based on an assessment of the current pipeline and the clinical success rates of these products (Food and Drug Administration, 2019b). According to the National Institutes of Health, 80% of rare diseases are caused by single-gene defects. CGTs, which are anticipated to treat the underlying causes of these genetic disorders, will play an ever-increasing role in treating rare diseases.

Although randomized, concurrent-controlled trials are still considered the gold standard for providing efficacy and safety data, they are often not feasible in trials of CGT for rare diseases. The combining characteristics of CGTs and rare diseases, including invasive procedures for administration, substantial unmet medical needs, and limited numbers of patients, require more flexibility for trial design (Food and Drug Administration, 2019a). A single-arm trial with an external control is often an option for CGTs and rare diseases, given appropriate natural history studies. In fact, among the approved CGT products by the FDA, the majority of them have been tested based on single-arm studies (Food and Drug Administration, 2021). Also, half of the CGT products approved by the EMA are only based on single-arm studies (Abou-El-Enein and Hey, 2019).

In the area of rare disease, natural history information is usually not available or is incomplete for most rare diseases; therefore, natural history study is particularly needed. A natural history study collects information about the natural history of a disease in the absence of an intervention, from the disease onset until either its resolution or the patient's death. Thus, natural history studies help researchers differentiate the improvement as the effect of the drug from the variations in the natural history of the disease or improvement resulting from the evolution of standard of care. Natural history studies can provide critical information for the selection of target patient populations and identification of clinical or surrogate endpoints. Moreover, if the patient population in the natural history studies is similar to the patient population receiving the drug, natural history studies can serve as the external controls for the evaluation of effectiveness and safety of drugs.

Zolgensma, initially approved by the FDA in 2019, is a gene therapy medication used to treat spinal muscular atrophy (SMA), a rare neuromuscular disorder considered as the most common genetic cause of infant death. Its approval was primarily based on two single-arm clinical trials using natural history studies as main comparator groups. The case study of Zolgensma will be helpful in providing deep insights on using natural history studies for CGT products to treat rare disease.

8.1.2 Spinal Muscular Atrophy

SMA with bi-allelic mutations in the *SMN1* gene is a rare, serious autosomal recessive neurodegenerative disorder. The clinical manifestations of SMA include progressive loss of muscle control, strength, and function; difficulty swallowing and breathing; and, ultimately, death. The main types of SMA are types 1, 2, 3, and 4 varying in the age of onset and clinical manifestations. SMA type 1 (also known as infantile-onset SMA) is the most severe and common form (approximately 45%–60%) of SMA. Patients with SMA type 1 show symptoms before 6 months of age and are never able to sit up, and most die of respiratory failure before reaching 2 years of age. SMA type 1 is the most common monogenic cause of infant mortality.

8.1.3 Natural History Studies of SMA

There are different types of natural history data available on SMA patients. Although patient registries and associated medical charts provided the sponsors of Zolgensma an initial understanding of the course of the disease, missing data or limited time course data restricted their use.

Two well-established natural history studies listed here provide a full picture of the natural history of SMA type 1 disease and therefore were used as external comparators by the sponsors for Zolgensma and the FDA.

Natural history study by Finkel et al. (2014).

- The study was a prospective cohort study that aimed to characterize the clinical features and course of SMA type 1. Patients were enrolled at three study sites and followed up for up to 36 months with serial clinical, motor function, laboratory, and electrophysiologic outcome assessments.
- The study enrolled a total of 34 SMA type 1 subjects.
- Key endpoints were ventilation-free survival, Children's Hospital of Philadelphia Infant Test for Neuromuscular Disorders (CHOP INTEND), and compound motor action potential (CMAP).
- Results: A total of 50% of these subjects completed at least 12 months of the follow-up. The median age reaching the combined endpoint of death or requiring at least 16 hours/day of ventilation support was 13.5 (interquartile range 8.1–22.0) months. The mean rate of decline in the CHOP INTEND motor function scale was 1.27 points/year (95% confidence interval 0.21–2.33, $p = 0.02$).

Natural history study by Kolb et al. (2017)

- The study was a longitudinal, multicenter, prospective natural history study on SMA type 1.
- The study enrolled a total of 26 SMA type 1 infants, and 27 healthy infants younger than 6 months as the control group.
- Key endpoints were permanent invasive ventilation-free survival, motor function scores (MFS), CMAP, and Test of Infant Motor Performance Screening Items.
- Results: MFS and CMAP decreased rapidly in SMA infants, whereas MFS in all healthy infants rapidly increased. Permanent invasive ventilation-free survival in SMA infants with two copies of survival of motor neuron 2 (SMN2) shows a median age of 8 months at death (95% confidence interval, 6, 17).

Although not referred by the FDA reviewers for Zolgensma, several other studies provided additional data on SMA type 1 natural history (De Sanctis et al., 2016; Kissel et al., 2011; Oskoui et al., 2007; Rudnik-Schöneborn et al., 2009). In summary, based on the natural history studies, the following conclusions were drawn:

- SMA type 1 patients never achieve sitting without support (De Sanctis et al., 2016; Finkel et al., 2014; Kolb et al., 2017).
- The rates of ventilation-free survival in SMA type 1 patients ranged from 9% to 51% at 18 months of age (Finkel et al., 2014; Kissel et al., 2011; Kolb et al., 2017; Oskoui et al., 2007; Rudnik-Schöneborn et al., 2009).
- Overall motor skills were assessed using the CHOP-INTEND score, which provides a standardized method of examining the movement

ability of infants. The CHOP-INTEND score is based on a question-naire that contains 16 items scored 0–4. The total score ranges from 0 to 64, and higher scores indicate better motor skills. None of the SMA type 1 infants with two copies of the SMN2 gene had an increase of at least 4 points from baseline in their CHOP-INTEND score after 12 months of follow-up.

8.1.4 Case Study of Zolgensma

8.1.4.1 Overview

Zolgensma is an adeno-associated virus vector-based gene therapy, where a single intravenous dose delivers a corrected copy of the *SMN1* gene to replace the non-functional or missing copy of the gene. All patients receiving the drug had baseline anti-adeno-associated virus 9 antibody titers of ≤1:50 and received oral corticosteroid to suppress potential immune reactions to the drug.

Zolgensma was approved by the FDA in 2019 for the treatment of pediatric patients younger than 2 years with SMA with bi-allelic mutations in the *SMN1* gene. Table 8.1.1 summarizes the five studies included in the biologics license applications submission.

The ongoing phase 3 clinical trial, AVXS-101-CL-303, and the completed phase 1 clinical trial, AVXS-101-CL-101, were the primary source of evidence for Zolgensma in patients younger than 2 years with SMA. The study AVXS-101-CL-303 provides the primary evidence of effectiveness, while AVXS-101-CL-101 provides supportive data. Data from additional ongoing

TABLE 8.1.1

Studies in the biologics license applications submission for Zolgensma

Study code	Study design	Study population	No. of subjects treated[a]	Status[a]
AVXS-101-CL-101	Phase 1, single center, single arm, single dose, dose escalation, IV trial	SMA type 1	15	Completed
AVXS-101-CL-102	Phase 1, U.S. multicenter, single dose, dose escalation, intrathecal trial	SMA type 2 and type 3	4	Ongoing
AVXS-101-CL-303	Phase 3, U.S. multicenter, single arm, single dose, IV trial	SMA type 1	12	Ongoing
AVXS-101-CL-304	Phase 3, global multicenter, single arm, single dose, IV presymptomatic trial	SMA type 1 and type 2	1	Ongoing
AVXS-101-LT-001	Long-term follow-up of patients from the AVXS-101-CL-101 study	SMA type 1	11	Ongoing

Source: FDA statistical review of Zolgensma Table 8.2.
[a] As of data cutoff date (May 8, 2018).

trials contribute further to the safety database. The FDA approval is based on improvement in permanent ventilation-free survival and achievement of developmental motor milestones such as sitting without support for ≥30 seconds. Permanent ventilation-free survival is defined as time to death or until the patient requires at least 16 hours per day of ventilation support for breathing for ≥14 consecutive days in the absence of an acute reversible illness, excluding perioperative use.

8.1.4.2 The AVXS-101-CL-303 Phase 3 Trial

The AVXS-101-CL-303 is an open-label, single-arm study. The trial enrolled 21 patients with infantile-onset SMA. All patients received the 1.1×10^{14} vg/kg dose. The study was ongoing at the time of regulatory submission.

There are two primary efficacy endpoints in the study:

1. Permanent ventilation-free survival at 14 months of age.
2. The proportion of patients achieving the milestone of sitting without support for at least 30 seconds at 18 months of age.

As of the March 2019 data cutoff, 19 patients were alive without the need for permanent ventilation (i.e., event-free survival) and continued in the trial; one patient withdrew from the study at age 11.9 months, and one patient died at age 7.8 months due to disease progression. The 19 surviving patients who were continuing in the trial ranged in age from 9.4 to 18.5 months. These patients were 7.9–15.4 months post-Zolgensma infusion. The results for survival and achievement of the milestone of sitting without support for ≥30 seconds are shown in Table 8.1.2. Comparison of the results of this study with available natural history data of infants with SMA provides primary evidence of the effectiveness of Zolgensma. In addition, 16 of the 19 patients had not required daily non-invasive ventilation use.

TABLE 8.1.2

Survival and motor milestone achievement in the ongoing phase 3 trial, the AVXS-101-CL-303 study

Endpoint	AVXS-101-CL-303 study ($N=21$) n (%)	Natural history study ($N=23$) %
Ventilation-free survival at 14 months of age[a]	13 (67%)	25%
Sitting without support for ≥30 seconds	10 (47%)	0

Source: FDA statistical review addendum of Zolgensma.
[a] Only 13 patients had reached 14 months of age by the data cutoff.

8.1.4.3 The AVXS-101-CL-101 Phase 1 Trial

The AVXS-101-CL-101 was an open-label, single-arm, ascending-dose study. The study enrolled a total of 15 infants with SMA. Two doses were evaluated in the trial. Three patients were enrolled in the low-dose 6.7×10^{13} vg/kg cohort, and 12 patients were enrolled in the high-dose 2.0×10^{14} vg/kg cohort. The key efficacy endpoints evaluated in the study AVXS-101-CL-101 are permanent ventilation-free survival, CHOP-INTEND from baseline, and achievement of significant development milestones. Comparison of the high-dose cohort with the low-dose cohort in terms of survival and motor milestone achievements at 24 months, as shown in Table 8.1.3, indicates a clear dose-response relationship of Zolgensma. Comparison of the results with the natural history studies of Finkel et al. (2014) and Kolb et al. (2017) provides further evidence of the effectiveness of Zolgensma.

8.1.5 Other Approved Drugs for SMA

In the area of SMA, two other drugs, Spinraza and Evrysdi, have been approved as of 2021. Spinraza, an antisense oligonucleotide drug that modifies the *SMN2* gene for producing more functional protein, is the first drug approved by the FDA to treat children and adults with SMA. Spinraza is delivered via intrathecal injection with four loading doses.

The sponsor once proposed to use the results from Finkel et al. (2014) as historical control to combine with a phase 2, open-label, dose-ranging study as the potential basis for an NDA. However, it was turned down by the FDA because of the confounding factors such as more intensive supportive care or differences in patient selection (Food and Drug Administration, 2017).

The FDA had multiple iterative interactions with the sponsor to help develop and refine its interim analysis plan for phase 3 (an ongoing double-blind, sham procedure-controlled trial). The result of the interim analysis of

TABLE 8.1.3

Survival and motor milestone achievement in the completed phase 1 trial, the AVXS-101-CL-101 study

Endpoint	Low-dose cohort ($N=3$)	High-dose cohort ($N=12$)	Natural history studies (%)
Permanent ventilation-free survival at 14 months of age	2 (67%)	12 (100%)	8%[a]
Sitting without support for ≥30 seconds	0	9 (75%)	0
Standing	0	2 (16.7%)	0[b]
Walking	0	2 (16.7%)	0[b]

Source: FDA statistical review of Zolgensma.

[a] Based on Kolb et al. (2017).
[b] Based on Finkel et al. (2014).

the phase 3 trial strongly supported the efficacy and led to the submission to the FDA.

Spinraza was ultimately approved in 2016 for the treatment of SMA in both pediatric and adult patients, mainly based on interim efficacy data from the double-blind phase 3 sham-controlled study.

Evrysdi, approved by the FDA in August 2020, is the first oral treatment for SMA patients aged 2 months or older. Similar to Spinraza, Evrysdi is designed to help the *SMN2* gene produce more functional SMN proteins.

The approval was based on two studies: Sunfish study—which enrolled patients with SMA type 2 or type 3 of 2–25 years of age, a randomized, double-blind, placebo-controlled study, and Firefish study—which enrolled patients with SMA type 1 of 1–7 months of age, an open-label, historical control study.

FDA reviewers acknowledged that the natural history of SMA is well understood. As a result, the natural history studies were used to interpret the results from the Firefish study focusing on SMA type 1 (De Sanctis et al., 2016; Finkel et al., 2014; Food and Drug Administration, 2020; Kolb et al., 2017).

8.1.6 Discussion

Natural history studies can potentially play a critical role in drug development, especially for rare diseases in various situations, such as identifying the target patient population, selecting clinical outcomes or biomarkers, and most importantly providing the source of alternative comparator groups. In the area of SMA, because there are well-established natural history studies and the outcome measures are objective and consistent with the clinical trials, it is possible to incorporate natural history studies as external control. In the case of Zolgensma, it was acknowledged by the FDA that

> Use of external historical controls, while not ideal, appears reasonable in this case, because an unmet medical need remain present for treatment of this fatal condition; the natural history of infantile-onset SMA is well-documented and follows a relatively predictable course that can be objectively measured and verified.
>
> *(Food and Drug Administration, 2019c)*

However, there are situations when it is difficult to use the natural history studies to interpret the clinical trial data. For example, in the case of Spinraza, the proposal of using natural history studies as historical control combining with a phase 2 study was turned down by the FDA due to comparability issues (lack of exchangeability). It was mentioned by an FDA reviewer that

> The sponsor asserted that the Phase 2 study results indicated a benefit on survival times and clinical assessments relative to natural history. However, confounding factors such as more intensive supportive care or differences in patient selection made them very difficult to interpret.
>
> *(Food and Drug Administration, 2017)*

There is increasing interest and acceptance from regulatory agencies to use natural history data for drug approval due to the availability of high-quality data from natural history studies. Borrowing information from external studies can not only be applied to single-arm studies but also to randomized controlled studies of small sample sizes. A classical reference to check exchangeability of data from natural history studies is Pocock's criteria (Pocock, 1976), which describe six necessary conditions for the external comparator group to be exchangeable with the randomized internal controls of a clinical trial.

References

Abou-El-Enein, M., & Hey, S. P. (2019). Cell and gene therapy trials: Are we facing an "evidence crisis"? *EClinicalMedicine*, *7*, 13–14. https://doi.org/10.1016/j.eclinm.2019.01.015

De Sanctis, R., Coratti, G., Pasternak, A., Montes, J., Pane, M., Mazzone, E. S., Young, S. D., Salazar, R., Quigley, J., Pera, M. C., Antonaci, L., Lapenta, L., Glanzman, A. M., Tiziano, D., Muntoni, F., Darras, B. T., De Vivo, D. C., Finkel, R., & Mercuri, E. (2016). Developmental milestones in type I spinal muscular atrophy. *Neuromuscular Disorders*, *26*(11), 754–759. https://doi.org/10.1016/j.nmd.2016.10.002

Finkel, R. S., McDermott, M. P., Kaufmann, P., Darras, B. T., Chung, W. K., Sproule, D. M., Kang, P. B., Foley, A. R., Yang, M. L., Martens, W. B., Oskoui, M., Glanzman, A. M., Flickinger, J., Montes, J., Dunaway, S., O'Hagen, J., Quigley, J., Riley, S., Benton, M., ... & De Vivo, D. C. (2014). Observational study of spinal muscular atrophy type I and implications for clinical trials. *Neurology*, *83*(9), 810–817. https://doi.org/10.1212/WNL.0000000000000741

Food and Drug Administration. (2017). *Spinraza (nusinersen) Medical Review(s)*. https://www.accessdata.fda.gov/drugsatfda_docs/nda/2016/209531Orig1s000MedR.pdf

Food and Drug Administration. (2019a). *FDA Guidance for Industry: Demonstrating Substantial Evidence of Effectiveness for Human Drug and Biological Products.* https://www.fda.gov/media/133660/download

Food and Drug Administration. (2019b). Statement from FDA Commissioner Scott Gottlieb, M.D. and Peter Marks, M.D., Ph.D., Director of the Center for Biologics Evaluation and Research on new policies to advance development of safe and effective cell and gene therapies. https://www.fda.gov/news-events/press-announcements/statement-fda-commissioner-scott-gottlieb-md-and-peter-marks-md-phd-director-center-biologics

Food and Drug Administration. (2019c). *ZOLGENSMA*. https://www.fda.gov/vaccines-blood-biologics/zolgensma

Food and Drug Administration. (2020). *Risdiplam Summary Review*. https://www.accessdata.fda.gov/drugsatfda_docs/nda/2020/213535Orig1s000SumR.pdf

Food and Drug Administration. (2021). *Approved Cellular and Gene Therapy Products.* https://www.fda.gov/vaccines-blood-biologics/cellular-gene-therapy-products/approved-cellular-and-gene-therapy-products

Kissel, J. T., Scott, C. B., Reyna, S. P., Crawford, T. O., Simard, L. R., Krosschell, K. J., Acsadi, G., Elsheik, B., Schroth, M. K., D'Anjou, G., LaSalle, B., Prior, T. W., Sorenson, S., Maczulski, J. A., Bromberg, M. B., Chan, G. M., & Swoboda, K. J. (2011). SMA carni-VAL trial part II: A prospective, single-armed trial of L-carnitine and valproic acid in ambulatory children with spinal muscular atrophy. *PLoS One, 6*(7), e21296. https://doi.org/10.1371/journal.pone.0021296

Kolb, S. J., Coffey, C. S., Yankey, J. W., Krosschell, K., Arnold, W. D., Rutkove, S. B., Swoboda, K. J., Reyna, S. P., Sakonju, A., Darras, B. T., Shell, R., Kuntz, N., Castro, D., Parsons, J., Connolly, A. M., Chiriboga, C. A., McDonald, C., Burnette, W. B., Werner, K., ... & Kissel, J. T. (2017). Natural history of infantile-onset spinal muscular atrophy. *Annals of Neurology, 82*(6), 883–891. https://doi.org/10.1002/ana.25101

Oskoui, M., Levy, G., Garland, C. J., Gray, J. M., O'Hagen, J., De Vivo, D. C., & Kaufmann, P. (2007). The changing natural history of spinal muscular atrophy type 1. *Neurology, 69*(20), 1931–1936. https://doi.org/10.1212/01.wnl.0000290830.40544.b9

Pocock, S. J. (1976). The combination of randomized and historical controls in clinical trials. *Journal of Chronic Diseases, 29*(3), 175–188. https://doi.org/10.1016/0021-9681(76)90044-8

Rudnik-Schöneborn, S., Berg, C., Zerres, K., Betzler, C., Grimm, T., Eggermann, T., Eggermann, K., Wirth, R., Wirth, B., & Heller, R. (2009). Genotype-phenotype studies in infantile spinal muscular atrophy (SMA) type I in Germany: Implications for clinical trials and genetic counselling. *Clinical Genetics, 76*(2), 168–178. https://doi.org/10.1111/j.1399-0004.2009.01200.x

---

8.2 Use of Electronic Health Records for Drug Approval: A Case Study of Xpovio® (Selinexor)

Chenkun Wang
Vertex Pharmaceuticals

8.2.1 Background

For several decades, randomized clinical trials have been the gold standard for generating efficacy evidence for drug products prior to the marketing authorization. In recent years, the rapid growth of computing technology promotes real-world data (RWD) to play an ever-increasing role in regulatory decision-making on drug products. By definition, RWD are routinely collected data of patients' health status or the delivery of health care from a variety of sources that is beyond conventional clinical trials, such as electronic health records (EHRs), medical claims, product and disease registries, laboratory test results, and data gathered from other sources that can inform on health status, such as mobile devices.

In certain cases, the data collected from RWD sources can be used in the analysis infrastructure to support many types of study designs to develop real-world evidence (RWE). The FDA has a long history of using RWE to monitor and evaluate the safety of drug products in post-marketing settings. However, the use of RWE to support effectiveness determinations is much more limited, primarily in the setting of oncology and rare diseases with significant unmet medical needs (Food and Drug Administration, 2018). Given the increasing interest in the use of RWD to support regulatory decision-making, Winona R. Bolislis et al. analyzed 27 case studies where RWD were applied in the regulatory approval between the years 1998 and 2019 (Bolislis et al., 2020). Among the case studies, the most common sources of RWD have been health or medical records (16 cases).

EHRs are used to the systematically collect and store patients' health information in a digital format, including a wide range of data, such as demographics, medical history, medication and allergies, immunization status, laboratory test results, radiology images, vital signs, personal statistics like age and weight, and billing information. EHRs offer the possibility to generate efficacy evidence for new medicines, competing with data from clinical trial settings; however, its heterogeneous nature brings challenges to data analysis. To understand the common challenges and pitfalls of the use of EHRs for regulatory decision-making, a closer look into the case of Xpovio® (selinexor) would be useful.

8.2.2 Case Study of Xpovio® (Selinexor)

Xpovio® (selinexor) was initially approved under accelerated approval for the treatment of adult patients with relapsed or refractory multiple myeloma (RRMM) who have received at least four prior therapies and whose disease is refractory to at least two proteasome inhibitors, at least two immunomodulatory agents, and an anti-CD38 monoclonal antibody.

Multiple myeloma is a rare cancer that forms in a type of white blood cell called plasma cell. Normal plasma cells are found in the bone marrow and help fight infections by making antibodies that recognize and attack germs. However, for patients with multiple myeloma, cancerous plasma cells accumulate out of control in the bone marrow and invade healthy blood cells. In 2019, over 32,000 individuals in the United States were diagnosed with this disease. It is believed that approximately 100,000 Americans currently have the disease.

The pivotal clinical trials and the supportive clinical trials for Xpovio new drug application (NDA) are summarized in Table 8.2.1.

The efficacy of Xpovio plus dexamethasone was evaluated in the pivotal study STORM Part 2 (NCT02336815), a multicenter, single-arm, open-label study of adults with relapsed or refractory multiple myeloma. The primary endpoint of the STORM study is the overall response rate, assessed by an Independent Review Committee based on the International Myeloma Working Group

TABLE 8.2.1

Pivotal and supportive clinical trials relevant to Xpovio NDA

Trial	Design	Population	Primary endpoint
Pivotal			
KCP-330-012 (STORM) Part 2	Phase 2b, open-label, single-arm study	Tripe-class refractory multiple myeloma (N=123)	Overall response rate
Supportive			
KCP-330-012 (STORM) Part 1	Phase 2b, open-label, single-arm study	Tripe- or double-class refractory multiple myeloma (N=79)	Overall response rate
KCP-330–001	Phase 1, dose escalation and dose expansion study	Advanced hematologic malignancies (N=286; MM N=81)	Safety and tolerability
KS-50039	Retrospective observational study using RWD	Flatiron Health Analytic Database (N=64)	OS

Source: Xpovio NDA/BLA Multi-disciplinary Review and Evaluation Table 13.

　　Triple-class refractory: if it is resistant to all three classes of standard myeloma therapies: proteasome inhibitors, immunomodulatory agents, and monoclonal antibodies.

OS, overall survival.

Uniform Response Criteria for Multiple Myeloma. The accelerated approval of Xpovio was mainly based on the efficacy and safety in a pre-specified subgroup analysis of 83 patients in STORM Part 2 whose disease was refractory to bortezomib, carfilzomib, lenalidomide, pomalidomide, and daratumumab as the benefit-to-risk ratio appeared to be greater in this more heavily pretreated population than in the overall trial population.

　　Among the supportive studies, the study KS-50039 was a retrospective observational study using EHR data from the Flatiron Health Analytic Database (FHAD). The FHAD is an oncology platform that aggregates EHR data from patients within the Flatiron network, which provides real-world clinical data collected from EHRs used by cancer care providers, including community and academic cancer centers, across the United States. An attrition diagram for selection of patients in the FHAD is provided in the Xpovio's NDA/BLA multidisciplinary review and evaluation, starting with 38,679 patients in the FHAD and ending up with 64 patients in the analysis (Food and Drug Administration, 2018b). The goals of the study KS-50039 is to compare the overall survival (OS) of the real-world cohort from the FHAD to the OS of the clinical trial cohort from STORM Part 2. However, the evidence generated from the study KS-50039 was challenged by the FDA and concluded that the comparison of survival between the FHAD and STORM is not appropriate. Examples of several key issues identified by the FDA are summarized as follows.

8.2.2.1 Biases or Issues Identified

8.2.2.1.1 Lack of Proof on Pre-Specified Analysis

To strengthen the trial integrity and enhance the transparency, the FDA expects to review and consent to study protocols or analysis plans prior to the initiation of study. However, in the submission of Xpovio, the FDA was made aware of the study KS-50039 on receiving the final study report. Therefore, the FDA cannot ensure that the analyses were pre-specified and unchanged during the study (Food and Drug Administration, 2018b).

8.2.2.1.2 Selection Bias

Substantial differences in the inclusion and exclusion criteria between the STORM and FHAD cohorts were likely to introduce selection bias. The criteria used to identify patients for STORM and the FHAD analysis were summarized and compared side by side in FDA's review. For example, an exclusion criterion for minimal life expectancy was not implemented for the FHAD population. Specifically, patients with less than 4 months of life expectancy were excluded from STORM; by contrast, no similar criteria were applied for the FHAD population so that the real-world OS of patients penta-exposed (patients have received lenalidomide, pomalidomide, bortezomib, carfilzomib, and daratumumab), triple-class refractory MM is 3.5–3.7 months. Such difference in selection criteria between the study arms systematically ensured that the STORM cohort was healthier and would have longer expected OS than the FHAD cohort (Food and Drug Administration, 2019).

8.2.2.1.3 Comparability Issue

In addition to the difference in inclusion and exclusion criteria, additional factors result in a lack of comparability between the FHAD and STORM cohorts. Imbalances in selected baseline characteristics between the FHAD and STORM cohorts were also noted. For example, differences in prior treatment histories and the distributions of Eastern Cooperative Oncology Group scores were observed. Moreover, the differences at baseline cannot be fully addressed due to incomplete baseline covariate data. For instance, baseline laboratory or comorbidity data were not available, and the baseline tumor stage status was mostly unknown in the FHAD cohort (Food and Drug Administration, 2019).

8.2.2.1.4 Index Date Issues

In clinical trials, the index date is usually defined as the date when patients receive their first study treatment. The primary endpoint of the study KS-50039 is to compare the OS, which is defined as the time from the index date to death by any cause. Therefore, the definition of the index date has a direct impact on the primary endpoint. The idea of index date was to set up date upon which a patient failed his or her last treatment and the dates originally defined as follows:

- FHAD: The end date of the regimen for which the patient's MM may first be defined as penta-exposed
- STORM: The progression date of the last line of therapy prior to Xpovio initiation for STORM patients who were penta-exposed, triple-class refractory

Such definition indicated that FHAD patients were indexed on the day when they became penta-exposed, but not necessarily on the day when they became triple-class refractory; thus, the date could be earlier than the date when the patient became triple-class refractory. During a later meeting with the applicant, the FDA requested an updated index date definition as the day of study treatment initiation after becoming penta-exposed and triple-class refractory for both STORM and FHAD cohorts (Food and Drug Administration, 2018b).

Additionally, the time elapsed from the start of the recruitment process to the start of drug therapy is usually considered immortal because patients must stay alive before the drug is administered. In clinical trials, the delays to starting treatment are generally short. However, immortal time bias can be problematic in external controls specifically in disease settings wherein mortality rates are high if index date definitions are not closely aligned (Burcu et al., 2020). According to the aforementioned definition, to set the index date for patients in STORM, one must look back into the patients record to determine the failure date of the previous regimen, resulting in excluding patients who do not live long enough to enroll in STORM. By contrast, patients with short survival times were not systematically excluded from the FHAD.

8.2.2.2 Additional Analyses Recommended

To address the issues identified for the study KS-50039, additional analyses were requested by the FDA.

For lack of comparability, the FDA encouraged the applicant to reconsider the eligibility criteria in the FHAD population as the original criteria identified patients different from the STORM population in key aspects and may bias the outcome in favor of the STORM population. Regarding the immortal time bias, the FDA requested the index date for the STORM patients to be defined as the start date of Xpovio initiation, or as the start date of the next treatment after becoming penta-exposed and triple-class refractory in the FHAD.

Although the applicant updated the analyses per FDA recommendation, evidence of incomparability across baseline characteristics persisted. Eventually, it was concluded that the evidence generated from the RWD analysis was not adequate to provide context or comparison for the OS observed in the STORM patients. Furthermore, FDA analysis found that post hoc strategies to create greater comparability across cohorts were inadequate and resulted in very limited sample size and unstable estimates (Food and Drug Administration, 2019).

8.2.3 Discussion

As previously stated, the FDA has used RWD primarily for the evaluation of safety monitoring. With an increasing interest of employing RWD to generate efficacy evidence of drug products, FDA's RWE Program has been working with stakeholders to explore the potential of RWD/RWE to support regulatory approval (Food and Drug Administration, 2018a).

One major use of RWD to support regulatory decision on drug effectiveness is to serve as an external control arm to enhance data from the single-arm trial (Bolislis et al., 2020), especially in the area of rare disease due to the limited patient population and/or the unmet medical need (Jahanshahi et al., 2021). However, using RWD as the basis for external controls has natural limitations, such as difficulties in selecting a comparable population, lack of standardized diagnostic criteria or equivalent outcome measures, and variability in follow-up procedures. EHRs, as one of the major sources for RWD, can provide data at the individual level, making possibilities for more comprehensive statistical analysis to reduce the biases.

Given the regulatory history, there are drug products initially approved using EHRs as external control, where the intrinsic limitations have been well minimized. For example, Blincyto® (blinatumomab) was initially approved under accelerated approval for the treatment of Philadelphia chromosome-negative relapsed or refractory B-cell precursor acute lymphoblastic leukemia, based on evidence of complete remission and duration of complete remission from a single-arm trial, the response rate of which was compared to historical data from 694 comparable patients extracted from over 2,000 patient records from the European Union and U.S. clinical study and treatment sites (Przepiorka et al., 2015).

There were cases where RWD study was part of the original NDA intended to provide supportive efficacy evidence, but the evidence from RWD was not considered sufficient by agency. Studying the issues found and the corresponding recommendations made by agency would be very helpful to understand agency's expectation on RWD study. In this section, the deep dive into the case study of Xpovio provides such a great opportunity to learn the insights into the use of RWD from agency's perspective.

References

Bolislis, W. R., Fay, M., & Kühler, T. C. (2020). Use of real-world data for new drug applications and line extensions. *Clinical Therapeutics*, 42(5), 926–938. https://doi.org/10.1016/j.clinthera.2020.03.006

Burcu, M., Dreyer, N. A., Franklin, J. M., Blum, M. D., Critchlow, C. W., Perfetto, E. M., & Zhou, W. (2020). Real-world evidence to support regulatory decision-making for medicines: Considerations for external control arms. *Pharmacoepidemiology and Drug Safety*, 29(10), 1228–1235. https://doi.org/https://doi.org/10.1002/pds.4975

Food and Drug Administration. (2018a). *Framework for FDA's Real-World Evidence Program*. https://www.fda.gov/media/120060/download

Food and Drug Administration. (2018b). *XPOVIO (Selinexor) Multi-Discipline Review*. https://www.accessdata.fda.gov/drugsatfda_docs/nda/2019/212306Orig1s000MultidisciplineR.pdf

Food and Drug Administration. (2019). *Drug Approval Package: XPOVIO*. https://www.accessdata.fda.gov/drugsatfda_docs/nda/2019/212306Orig1s000TOC.cfm

Jahanshahi, M., Gregg, K., Davis, G., Ndu, A., Miller, V., Vockley, J., Ollivier, C., Franolic, T., & Sakai, S. (2021). The use of external controls in FDA regulatory decision making. *Therapeutic Innovation & Regulatory Science*. https://doi.org/10.1007/s43441-021-00302-y

Przepiorka, D., Ko, C.-W., Deisseroth, A., Yancey, C. L., Candau-Chacon, R., Chiu, H.-J., Gehrke, B. J., Gomez-Broughton, C., Kane, R. C., Kirshner, S., Mehrotra, N., Ricks, T. K., Schmiel, D., Song, P., Zhao, P., Zhou, Q., Farrell, A. T., & Pazdur, R. (2015). FDA approval: Blinatumomab. *Clinical Cancer Research*, 21(18), 4035–4039. https://doi.org/10.1158/1078-0432.CCR-15-0612

8.3 Use of Basket Trial: A Case Study of VITRAKVI® (Larotrectinib)

Tu Xu
Vertex Pharmaceuticals

8.3.1 Background

The conventional drug development process typically consists of multiple RCTs that evaluate individual disease indications for one investigational product. The corresponding evidence generated is considered to demonstrate the effectiveness of investigational products of high quality. However, the conventional approach becomes infeasible and cost-ineffective for medical research on rare diseases with high unmet medical needs. One emerging solution is to utilize clinical trials with master protocols (Woodcock and LaVange, 2017; Berry et al., 2015). The master protocol concept is to provide a platform for simultaneously evaluating multiple agents (umbrella trials) or disease indications (basket trials) (Figure 8.3.1) with the goal of increasing operational efficiency, and to accelerate the drug development process.

In the past two decades, therapies that target specific disease-causing genetic variability have led to multiple brilliant medical breakthroughs, especially in the oncology area. One amazing characteristic of target therapies

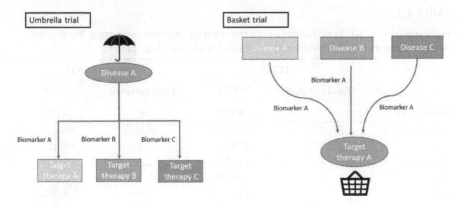

FIGURE 8.3.1
Umbrella trials and basket trials.

is that some target therapies could work well across cancer types caused by the same genetic disorder. The most well-known example is pembrolizumab (Keytruda), an immune checkpoint inhibitor of PD-1. Pembrolizumab shows unprecedent treatment benefits in RCTs for a variety of solid tumors. However, in some cases, the extremely low prevalence of targeted genes would make RCTs infeasible for evaluating new therapies. Since transformative treatment benefits are present consistently across indications driven by target gene, basket trial design becomes an ideal option to consolidate the investigation on multiple rare indications into one study to facilitate the development process. Recently, there are successful applications of master protocol that accelerated the clinical development of targeted therapies (Chen et al., 2016, Drilon et al., 2018). For example, larotrectinib received unprecedent tissue-agnostic approvals from the FDA and EMA based on a pivotal basket study. These approvals allow larotrectinib to treat all solid tumors with *NTKR* gene fusions, which endure high unmet medical needs, while the prevalence is <1% in common solid tumor types.

8.3.2 Case Study on Tissue-Agnostic Type Approval

8.3.2.1 Larotrectinib

8.3.2.1.1 Evidence to Support Regulatory Approvals

Larotrectinib (VITRAKVI) is a kinase inhibitor developed by Loxo Oncology that targets the *NTRK* gene fusion and inhibits the kinase activities of the tropomyosin receptor kinases *TRKA, TRKB,* and *TRKC* (Drilon et al., 2018). It is discovered that TRK fusions lead to oncogene addition, regardless of types of solid tumors. Although the *NTRK* gene fusion is frequently observed in some extremely rare cancers (e.g., >90% for secretory breast carcinoma), the NTRK gene fusions are generally rare (<1%), with low frequencies reported for most common cancer types (Table 8.3.1).

TABLE 8.3.1

Frequency of NTRK gene fusion in common types of cancers (Europe Medicines Agency, Committee for Medicinal Products for Human Use, 2019)

	TCGA		Project GENIE	
	Total samples	NTRK	Total samples	NTRK
Tumor type	*N*	*n* (%)	*N*	*n* (%)
All tumor types	5221	35(0.67%)	41,882	83 (0.2%)
NSCLC	517	1 (0.19%)	8,559	9 (0.11%)
Melanoma	468	1 (0.21%)	2,291	5 (0.21%)
CRC	557	3 (0.54%)	5,795	7 (0.12%)
Pancreas	178	2 (1.12%)	1,966	5 (0.25%)
Breast cancer	1026	2 (0.19%)	8,075	9 (0.11%)

TABLE 8.3.2

Clinical studies supporting the safety and efficacy of larotrectinib

Study	Study design
LOXO-TRK-14001	Open-label, 3+3 dose escalation, adult patients, advanced solid tumors
LOXO-TRK-15001	Open-label basket trial, 12 years of age or older with NTRK fusion advanced cancer
LOXO-TRK-15003	Open-label, dose escalation study, pediatric patients with advanced solid, or primary CNS tumors

Due to the extreme rarity of *NTRK* gene fusions, regulatory agencies agreed that it is infeasible to conduct randomized trials in patients with *NTRK*-positive solid tumors. Given the strong biologic rational and preclinical data on larotrectinib activity across tumor types, the FDA accepted using data from three single-arm clinical studies to support the clinical assessments of safety and efficacy of larotrectinib (Table 8.3.2).

The primary efficacy endpoint is the overall response rate (ORR), and the secondary endpoint is the duration of response (DOR). As aligned between Loxo Oncology and the FDA, a treatment with a true ORR of 30% or more is considered effective. The primary efficacy analysis was to be conducted based on the first 55 patients with *NTRK* fusion solid tumors enrolled in three clinical studies. Assume a true ORR of at least 50%, a sample size of 55 could provide 80% power to rule out 30% from the lower bound of two-sided 95% confidence interval of ORR.

For the 55 patients included in primary efficacy analysis, 35 of these patients were enrolled in the pivotal single-arm phase 2 study (LOXO-TRK 15002). The LOXO-TRK 15002 study adopts a basket trial design including nine cohorts of patients with a variety of solid tumors bearing NTRK gene fusion (see Figure 8.3.2). The remaining 20 patients were enrolled in LOXO-TRK 14001 (*N* = 8) and LOXO-TRK 15003 (*N* = 12).

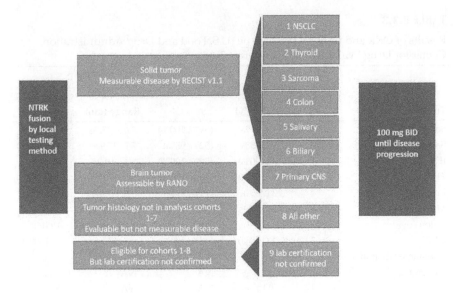

FIGURE 8.3.2
Study design of LOXO-TRK 15002. (U.S. Food and Drug Administration, Center for Drug Evaluation and Research, 2018.)

Supported by the strong scientific rational (non-clinical and clinical) that tumor shrinkage due to the inhibition of TRK is consistent in tumors with *NTRK* gene fusions, the primary efficacy analysis was conducted by pooling the data of these 55 patients, although variability of tumor types and adult and pediatric populations is acknowledged. The initial analysis in July 2017 shown an ORR of 75% (95% CI: 61%, 85%), a complete response (CR) rate of 13%, and durable response to treatment (46% of DOR ≥6 months) according to the assessment of the independent radiology committee. FDA reviewers further conducted subgroup analyses by tumor types, and the results appear to be consistent (Table 8.3.3).

In November 2018, based on the strong non-clinical support and promising clinical data on efficacy and safety, the FDA granted accelerated approval to larotrectinib for treating adult and pediatric patients with solid tumors that carry *NTRK* gene fusions. This is the second tissue-agnostic type approval from the FDA after the approval of pembrolizumab for treating MSI-H/dMMR metastatic solid tumors.

Similarly, for the EU marketing authorization application of larotrectinib, the EMA agreed using data from single-arm studies (LOXO-TRK 14001, LOXO-TRK 15002, LOXO-TRK 15003) as a basis of evidence due to rarity of patients with *NTRK* gene fusions. In addition to the data of the first 55 subjects included in the FDA application, additional data from other patients with *NTRK* gene fusions enrolled in these three clinical studies (total $N=102$) were also provided. Consistent effectiveness in the ORR and DOR was observed. In July 2019, larotrectinib was granted a tissue-agnostic type

TABLE 8.3.3

Results of ORR and DOR by tumor type (U.S. Food and Drug Administration, Center for Drug Evaluation and Research, 2018)

Tumor type	Patient (*n*)	ORR		DOR	
		Rspn (%)	95% CI[a]	Range (mo)	≥ 6 months, n(%)
Soft tissue sarcoma	11	10 (91%)	(59%, 100%)	3.6+, 33.2+	7 (70%)
Salivary gland	12	10 (83%)	(52%, 98%)	7.7, 27.9+	10 (100%)
IFS	7	7 (100%)	(59%, 100%)	1.4+,10.2+	2 (33%)
Thyroid	5	5 (100%)	(48%, 100%)	3.7, 27.0+	4 (80%)
Lung	4	3 (75%)	(19%, 99%)	8.2, 20.3+	3 (100%)
Melanoma	4	2 (50%)	NA	1.9+, 17.5+	1 (50%)
Colon	4	1 (25%)	NA	5.6	1 (100%)
GIST	3	3 (100%)	(29%, 100%)	9.5, 17.3	3 (100%)
Cholangiocarcinoma	2	SD, NE	NA	NA	NA
Appendix	1	SD	NA	NA	NA
Breast	1	PD	NA	NA	NA
Pancreas	1	SD	NA	NA	NA

[1] Observed values at data cutoff, not a range. Data cutoff date: February 19, 2018.
CR, complete response; NA, not applicable; PD, progression disease; PR, partial response; Rspn, responder number; SD, stable disease.
[a] No 95% CI for less than three responders.

marketing authorization by the EMA for treating patients with solid tumors bearing *NTRK* gene fusion. This was the first histology-independent treatment approved by the EMA.

8.3.2.1.2 Regulatory Considerations on Statistical Analyses

Although larotrectinib shows favorable efficacy in pooled analysis and subgroup analyses by tumor type, regulatory agencies expressed concerns regarding the uncertainty on the magnitude of the treatment effect across tumor types. The efficacy summary based on a simple pooling strategy may provide a biased characterization of the clinical benefit of larotrectinib for each tumor type.

As outlined in the FDA review report (2018),

> FDA accepted data pooled from 3 single arm trials due to the extreme rarity of NTRK fusion positive solid tumors, rendering conduct of a randomized trial infeasible...each with different natural histories, "lumping" all tumor types together into a single randomized trial would present significant challenges in trial design and analysis of the data...

The EMA review report (2019) also pointed out that the efficacy data presented were not considered comprehensive, and the benefit in subgroups of patients based on histology needs to be further studied.

As more precise estimates of efficacy in those common histologic tumor types were essential, both the FDA and EMA requested Loxo Oncology to enroll additional patients and conduct long-term follow-ups as the post-marketing requirements to verify and characterize the clinical benefit of larotrectinib.

In the literature, there has been extensive research conducted to address heterogeneity across indications. Adaptive pooling strategies are well known with the objective of pooling information only from patients with homogenous outcomes. Bayesian adaptive borrowing strategies were proposed (Ibrahim and Chen, 2000; Hobbs et al., 2011; Chu and Yuan, 2018) to allow flexible information borrowing for analyses. Chen et al. (2016) proposed an innovative basket trial design that prunes the inactive indications at an interim analysis and then pools the active indications in the final analysis.

8.3.2.2 *Other Tissue-Agnostic Approvals*

Pembrolizumab (Keytruda) is a targeted therapy of PD-1 blocking antibody. In May 2017, the FDA granted accelerated approval to pembrolizumab for adult and pediatric patients with unresectable or metastatic, microsatellite instability-high (MSI-H) or mismatch repair-deficient (dMMR) solid tumors. Prior to that, pembrolizumab was approved to treat a variety of common cancer indications based on evidence from RCTs.

It was discovered that dMMR or MSI-H are sensitive to PD-1 inhibitor, regardless of tumor location and tumor type. The new drug application is primarily based on data of 149 subjects identified with MSI-H or dMMR tumor status (15 tumor types) from five single-arm clinical trials. This approval is based on clinical data of 149 patients with a variety of MSI-H or dMMR cancers from five non-randomized clinical trials, including the basket study KEYNOTE-158 with rare tumor cohorts. An ORR of 38% and durable response were observed in the analysis of the 149 subjects. It is the first tissue-agnostic type approval of the FDA.

Entrectinib (Rozlytrek) is an inhibitor of ROS proto-oncogene 1 receptor tyrosine kinase (encoded by the ROS1 gene); tropomyosin receptor kinases A, B, and C (TRKA, TRKB, and TRKC); and anaplastic lymphoma kinase (ALK). Similar to larotrectinib, the new drug application of entrectinib was based on data of 54 adult patients with NTRK-positive tumors from three single-arm clinical trials (ALKA $n=1$, STARTRK-1 $n=2$, and STARTRK-2 $n=51$), and STARTRK-2 is a phase 2 basket study with patients assigned to different cohorts according to tumor type. The primary endpoints are ORR and DOR. The analysis based on the 54 patients yielded an ORR of 57.4%, a CR rate of 7%, and durable response to treatment (55% of DOR≥6 months). In August 2019, the FDA granted tissue-agnostic approval to entrectinib for adults and pediatric patients 12 years of age and older with solid tumor harboring NTRK gene fusion. It marks the third tissue-agnostic approval by the FDA. In June 2020, entrectinib was approved by the EMA for the same indication, which becomes the second tissue-agnostic approval from the EMA following the approval of larotrectinib.

8.3.3 Summary and Discussion

In the past few decades, target therapies developed with strong biological rational have demonstrated transformative clinical benefits to address high unmet medical needs for a group of patients carrying specific genetic variation. When the target disease population is rare, traditional RCTs are no longer feasible for clinical development of those therapies. The emerging platform trial idea provides an exciting option to boost clinical development efficiency such that those transformative medications can become available to patients at an earlier time.

It is encouraging to observe the increased use of platform study design by sponsors and more support and guidance from regulatory agencies. Although uncertainty of evidence generated by the platform trial is still a concern, it has attracted broad interest from industry, regulatory, and academia in developing strategies to alleviate the risk, such as by using real-world evidence. The future of platform trials for clinical development of rare diseases looks promising.

References

Berry, S., Broglio, K., Groshen, S., and Berry, D. (2013) Bayesian hierarchical modelling of patient subpopulation: efficient designs of Phase II oncology clinical trials, *Clinical Trials*, **10**: 720–734.

Berry, S., Connor, J., and Lewis, R. (2015), The platform trial: an efficient strategy for evaluating multiple treatments, *The Journal of the American Medical Association*, **313**: 16.

Chen, C., Li, X., Yuan, S. and et al. (2016) Statistical design and considerations of a Phase 3 basket trial for simultaneous investigation of multiple tumor types in one study, *Statistics in Biopharmaceutical Research*, **8**: 248–257.

Chen, M., Ibrahim, J. (2000) Power prior distributions for regression models, *Statistical Science*, **15**: 46–60

Chu, Y., Yuan, Y. (2018) A Bayesian basket trial design using a calibrated Bayesian hierarchical model, *Clinical Trial*, **15**: 149–158.

Drilon A., Laetsch T., Kummar, S., and et al. (2018) Efficacy of larotrectinib in TRK fusion–positive cancers in adults and children, *New England Journal of Medicine*, **378**: 731–739.

Europe Medicines Agency, Committee for Medicinal Products for Human Use (2019) VITRAKVI assessment report, July 25, 2019. https://www.ema.europa.eu/en/documents/assessment-report/vitrakvi-epar-public-assessment-report_en.pdf

Hobbs, B., Carlin, B., Mandrekar, S., and Sargent, D. (2011) Hierarchical commensurate and power prior models for adaptive incorporation of historical information in clinical trials, *Biometrics*, **67**: 1047–1056.

U.S. Food and Drug Administration, Center for Drug Evaluation and Research (2018) VITRAKVI (larotrectinib) NDA multidisciplinary review and evaluation, November 26, 2018. https://www.accessdata.fda.gov/drugsatfda_docs/nda/2019/212725Orig1s000,%20212726Orig1s000MultidisciplineR.pdf

Woodcock, J., and LaVange, L. (2017) Master protocols to study multiple therapies, multiple diseases, or both, *New England Journal of Medicine*, **377**: 62–70.

8.4 Use of Biomarker as Surrogate Endpoint for Accelerated Approval: A Case Study of VYONDYS 53 (Golodirsen)

Jason Yuan
Neumora Therapeutics

Tina Liu
Vertex Pharmaceuticals

8.4.1 Background about Accelerated Approval

The conventional drug development process typically consists of a series of clinical trials from phase 1 to phase 3. The phase 3 confirmatory study is to generate data evidence to sufficiently demonstrate the effect of investigational product and the safety profile. However, sometimes, a large confirmatory phase 3 study becomes challenging or impracticable to recruit enough patients on rare diseases. Therefore, regulatory agencies such as the FDA has rolled out accelerated approval for such cases, especially for serious conditions with high unmet medical needs (FDA Guidance for Industry, 2014). Under such programs by regulatory agencies, the drug development sponsors are allowed to submit the data evidence generated from phase ½ studies using surrogate or intermediate clinical endpoints for accelerated approval, instead of waiting for the phase 3 study results, which could take many years to finish. At the same time, the drug development sponsors will still be required to conduct and finish the phase 3 confirmatory trial as a regulatory commitment to confirm the clinical benefits of the new drug. If the phase 3 study does not show clinical benefit in the end, the regulatory agency could withdraw the approval and remove the drug from market.

In the past two decades, the breakthrough of disease-targeted therapies and novel therapies (e.g., RNA, cell, and gene therapies) has led to the discovery of a series of new medicines and showed promising efficacy in early phase 1/2 studies based on biomarkers or surrogate endpoints. Quite a few of them received accelerated approvals by the FDA, especially in oncology and rare disease areas, where the medical unmet need is high. The accelerated approvals by the FDA have become an efficient and successful program to obtain the novel breakthrough medicines to meet patients' need, without additional long time waiting for the completion of the phase 3 confirmatory trial. For example, Velcade in multiple myeloma and Gleevec in chronic myeloid leukemia received accelerated approvals based on response rate results, instead of survival benefit based on similar considerations from the FDA (Velcade 2003 NDA approval letter; Gleevec 2001 NDA approval letter). These approvals have been well recognized by the medical society and patient associations. Recently, multiple successful applications of treatment for Duchenne muscular dystrophy (DMD) based on RNA technologies (e.g., EXONDYS 51, VYONDYS 53, AMONDYS 45, and VILTEPSO) were granted accelerated approvals by the FDA, which ensure high unmet medical needs for the children with DMD. These treatments shared similar mechanism targeting different locations of gene mutation. The accelerated approval of Exondys 51 set the precedence for the accelerated approvals of later therapies of the same class.

8.4.2 Case Study on Accelerated-Type Approvals Based on Biomarkers

8.4.2.1 VYONDYS 53 (Golodirsen)

8.4.2.1.1 Introduction of DMD and VYONDYS 53 (Golodirsen)

DMD affects one in 3,500–5,000 male children born worldwide (Foster et al., 2006, Crisafulli et al., 2020). It is a rare, fatal progressive neuromuscular genetic disease. The average lifespan of DMD patients is about mid to late 20s. The diagnosis typically occurs between ages 3 and 5 years. It was caused by gene mutation that encodes dystrophin, a protein that plays a key structural role in muscle fiber protection (Straub and Campbell, 1997). Certain mutation in dystrophin genes could stop the production of dystrophin protein. Exon skipping therapy is intended to address the underlying cause of disease by masking the error in the dystrophin gene, which allows for production of a shortened and potentially functional protein to support muscle function. Exon skipping therapy relies on the type and location of mutation on the dystrophin gene; thus, it targets only a subgroup of patients. Patients amenable to exon 51 and exon 53 skipping are estimated to comprise only 10%–14% of the total population, respectively. The population amenable to other exon skipping are even smaller: for example, 7%–9% amenable to exon 45 skipping and 4% to exon 6–7 (Magri et al., 2011, Bladen et al., 2015).

VYONDYS 53 (golodirsen) is an antisense oligonucleotide using Sarepta's proprietary phosphorodiamidate morpholino oligomer chemistry and exon skipping technology to bind to exon 53 of dystrophin pre-mRNA, resulting in exclusion, or "skipping," of this exon during mRNA processing in patients with genetic mutations that are amenable to exon 53 skipping.

8.4.2.1.2 Evidence to Support Regulatory Approvals of VYONDYS 53 (golodirsen)

Due to the rarity of DMD disease with many different types of mutations, it will take a very long time to complete a large randomized phase 3 study. Given the strong biologic rational and preclinical data on the biomarker of dystrophin and high unmet medical needs for these young children patients with DMD, the FDA accepted using the surrogate endpoint to support accelerated approval of VYONDYS 53 (golodirsen).

The effect of VYONDYS 53 on dystrophin production was evaluated in one phase 1/2 clinical study in DMD patients with a confirmed mutation of the DMD gene that is amenable to exon 53 skipping (FDA labeling for VYONDYS 53, 2019; NCT02310906). The study included two parts:

Part 1 was a double-blind, placebo-controlled, dose titration study in 12 DMD patients. The patients were randomized 2:1 to receive VYONDYS 53 or a matching placebo. The VYONDYS 53-treated patients received four escalating dose levels, ranging from 4 mg/kg/week (less than the recommended dosage) to 30 mg/kg/week by intravenous infusion for 2 weeks at each dose level.

Part 2 was a 168-week, open-label study assessing the efficacy and safety of VYONDYS 53 at a dose of 30 mg/kg/week in the 12 patients enrolled in part 1 plus 13 additional treatment-naive patients with DMD amenable to exon 53 skipping. At study entry (either in part 1 or in part 2), patients had a median age of 8 years and were on a stable dose of corticosteroids for at least 6 months. Efficacy was assessed based on change from baseline in the dystrophin protein level (measured as % of the dystrophin level relative to healthy subjects, i.e., % of normal) at week 48 of part 2. Muscle biopsies were obtained at baseline prior to treatment and at week 48 of part 2 in all VYONDYS 53-treated patients ($n=25$) and were analyzed for the dystrophin protein level by Western blot.

The dystrophin protein level was regarded as a surrogate endpoint that is reasonably likely to predict clinical benefit for DMD patients, and the accelerated approval was based on a statistically significant increase in dystrophin production: for the 25 patients treated by VYONDYS 53 in the study, the mean baseline dystrophin level (% relative to healthy subjects) was 0.10% (SD=0.07%). At week 48, the mean dystrophin level was 1.02% (SD=1.03%) for a mean increase of 0.92% (SD=1.01%) of normal levels ($p<0.001$). The median change from baseline was 0.88%.

In December 2019, based on the efficacy results of the dystrophin surrogate endpoint and safety data, the FDA granted accelerated approval to VYONDYS 53 (golodirsen) for the treatment of Duchenne muscular dystrophy (DMD) in patients amenable to skipping exon 53 (FDA accelerated approval letter for VYONDYS 53, 2019).

8.4.2.1.3 Regulatory Considerations and Post-Marketing Requirements on VYONDYS 53 (Golodirsen)

Although no clinical outcomes have demonstrated to have statistically significant effect at the time of submission, accelerated approval was considered based on the following considerations: (1) DMD clearly meets the criteria of a serious and life-threatening condition; (2) the safety profile of the drug was well tolerated with not much long-term concern; and (3) rare disease with limitation to perform a large-scale study in a reasonable time frame.

In addition, the FDA did provide several comments on the uncertainties of actual clinical benefit (FDA clinical review for VYONDYS 53, 2019):

- "There remains uncertainty regarding the level of dystrophin that would be likely to confer clinical benefit."
- "The correlation between the change in 6-minute walk distance (clinical benefit) and change in dystrophin (biomarker) is quite poor ($R = 0.14$)."
- "It seems likely that the clinical benefit associated with this change in dystrophin would be commensurately small. The clinical results of Study 4053-101 further suggest that if there is indeed an effect of golodirsen, the effect is small."

Therefore, the FDA imposed a post-marketing requirement for VYONDYS 53 (golodirsen) to complete a placebo-controlled, post-marketing confirmatory trial as a post-marketing requirement with the golodirsen arm to demonstrate a significant and clinically meaningful effect. Sarepta's placebo-controlled, post-marketing confirmatory trial, titled ESSENCE (NCT02500381), is carried out to support the VYONDYS 53 accelerated approval. Consistent with the accelerated approval pathway, the continued approval of VYONDYS 53 may be contingent on confirmation of a clinical benefit in this post-marketing confirmatory trial.

8.4.2.2 Other Accelerated Approvals by the FDA

In addition to VYONDYS 53 (golodirsen), the exon skipping therapies of the same mechanism of action have received accelerated approvals based on the same type of biomarker results:

- EXONDYS 51 (FDA accelerated approval letter for EXONDYS 51, 2016)
- AMONDYS 45 (FDA accelerated approval letter for Amondys 45, 2021)
- Viltepso (FDA accelerated approval letter for Viltepso, 2020)

Many novel oncology drugs also received accelerated approval based on response rates or other biomarkers as surrogate endpoints to predict survival benefit based on similar considerations from the FDA, such as Velcade in multiple myeloma (FDA accelerated approval letter for Velcade, 2003) and Gleevec in chronic myeloid leukemia (FDA accelerated approval letter for Gleevec, 2001).

The European Medicines Agency also supports a conditional marketing authorization (European Medicines Agency conditional marketing authorization, n.d.) for such medicines on less comprehensive clinical data than normally required, where the benefit of immediate availability of the medicine for unmet medical needs outweighs the risk inherent in the fact that additional data are still required. Medicines for human use are eligible if they are intended for treating, preventing, or diagnosing seriously debilitating or life-threatening diseases. This includes orphan medicine. Similarly, once a conditional marketing authorization has been granted, the marketing authorization holder must fulfil specific obligations within defined timelines.

8.4.3 Summary and Discussion

In the past few decades, it has been increasingly recognized that the phase 3 confirmatory study is important to generate data evidence to sufficiently demonstrate the effect of investigational product and the safety profile. However, new challenges are rising for novel clinical development as the targeted population could be extremely rare with high unmet medical needs. In this case, the conventional approach to evaluate the treatment benefit including a large phase 3 confirmatory study may not be feasible in a reasonable time frame to meet patients' needs. Therefore, regulatory agencies such the FDA has rolled out accelerated approval or conditional approval for such cases based on phase 1 and/or phase 2 data, especially for those with high unmet medical needs.

It is encouraging to observe the increased use of biomarkers in early phase studies by sponsors and accelerated approval support from regulatory agencies for breakthrough novel medicines. Although uncertainty of evidence generated by biomarkers in early phase studies is still a big challenge, it is encouraging to see rapid development of strategies to reduce the concerns, such as the use of real-world evidence and correlation between biomarkers and clinical benefit outcomes. The use of biomarkers for accelerated approval is expected to be more for rare diseases, along with the advancement of drug development technology and better use of real-world evidence data.

References

Bladen CL, Salgado D, Monges S, Foncuberta ME, Kekou K, Kosma K, Dawkins H, Lamont L, Roy AJ, Chamova T, Guergueltcheva V. The TREAT-NMD DMD global database: analysis of more than 7,000 Duchenne muscular dystrophy mutations. *Human Mutation.* 2015 Apr;36(4):395–402.

Crisafulli S, Sultana J, Fontana A, Salvo F, Messina S, Trifirò G. Global epidemiology of Duchenne muscular dystrophy: an updated systematic review and meta-analysis. *Orphanet Journal of Rare Diseases.* 2020 Dec;15(1):1–20.

EMA conditional marketing authorization, n.d. https://www.ema.europa.eu/en/human-regulatory/marketing-authorisation/conditional-marketing-authorisation

FDA accelerated approval letter for Amondys 45, 2021. https://www.accessdata.fda.gov/drugsatfda_docs/appletter/2021/213026Orig1s000ltr.pdf

FDA accelerated approval letter for EXONDYS 51, 2016. https://www.accessdata.fda.gov/drugsatfda_docs/appletter/2016/206488orig1s000ltr.pdf

FDA accelerated approval letter for Gleevec, 2001. https://www.accessdata.fda.gov/drugsatfda_docs/nda/2001/21-335_Gleevec_Approv.pdf

FDA accelerated approval letter for Velcade, 2003. https://www.accessdata.fda.gov/drugsatfda_docs/nda/2003/21602_Velcade_Approv.pdf

FDA accelerated approval letter for Viltepso, 2020. https://www.accessdata.fda.gov/drugsatfda_docs/appletter/2020/212154Orig1s000ltr.pdf

FDA accelerated approval letter for VYONDYS 53, 2019. https://www.accessdata.fda.gov/drugsatfda_docs/appletter/2019/211970Orig1s000ltr.pdf

FDA clinical review for VYONDYS 53, 2019. https://www.accessdata.fda.gov/drugsatfda_docs/nda/2019/211970Orig1s000MedR.pdf

FDA Guidance for Industry, 2014. Expedited programs for serious conditions – drugs and biologics. https://www.fda.gov/drugs/information-health-care-professionals-drugs/accelerated-approval-program

FDA Labelling for VYONDYS 53, 2019. https://www.accessdata.fda.gov/drugsatfda_docs/nda/2019/211970Orig1s000Lbl.pdf

Foster K, Foster H, Dickson JG. Gene therapy progress and prospects: Duchenne muscular dystrophy. *Gene Therapy*. 2006 Dec;13(24):1677–1685.

Magri F, Govoni A, D'Angelo MG, Del Bo R, Ghezzi S, Sandra G, … & Comi GP. Genotype and phenotype characterization in a large dystrophinopathic cohort with extended follow-up. *Journal of Neurology*. 2011;258(9):1610–1623.

Straub V, Campbell KP. Muscular dystrophies and the dystrophin-glycoprotein complex. *Current Opinion in Neurology*. 1997 Apr 1;10:168–175.

Index

Note: **Bold** page numbers refer to tables and *italic* page numbers refer to figures.

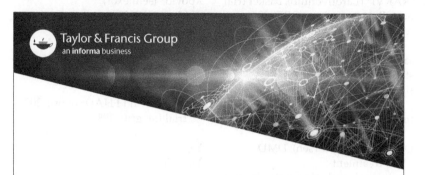

Taylor & Francis eBooks

www.taylorfrancis.com

A single destination for eBooks from Taylor & Francis
with increased functionality and an improved user
experience to meet the needs of our customers.

90,000+ eBooks of award-winning academic content in
Humanities, Social Science, Science, Technology, Engineering,
and Medical written by a global network of editors and authors.

TAYLOR & FRANCIS EBOOKS OFFERS:

A streamlined
experience for
our library
customers

A single point
of discovery
for all of our
eBook content

Improved
search and
discovery of
content at both
book and
chapter level

REQUEST A FREE TRIAL
support@taylorfrancis.com

Routledge
Taylor & Francis Group

CRC Press
Taylor & Francis Group